Schizophrenia

My Life after Being Diagnosed with Schizophrenia

Robert J. Burke

Copyright © 2022 Robert J. Burke
All rights reserved
First Edition

PAGE PUBLISHING
Conneaut Lake, PA

First originally published by Page Publishing 2022

ISBN 978-1-6624-8718-7 (pbk)
ISBN 978-1-6624-8724-8 (digital)

Printed in the United States of America

To my wonderful children, Allie and Jack
To my mom, Mary Ann; my deceased father Thomas C. Burke; my brothers Michael and Tommy; my beloved sisters Betsy, Eileen, and Mary Kay; my friends Deacon Tony, Fr. Neil, Fr. Bill, Fr. Tri, and the adept Dr. Arun Munjal.

Contents

Acknowledgment vii
Chapter 1: Introduction..1
Chapter 2: Life without Illness..8
Chapter 3: Diagnoses...14
Chapter 4: Troubles with Law Enforcement...............................25
Chapter 5: Sins and Forlorn..45
Chapter 6: Memories..50
Chapter 7: Rediscovery...61
Chapter 8: Schizophrenia—a Way Forward 72
Chapter 9: Lessons Learned 77

Acknowledgment

God the Almighty Father and Ignatius House

Chapter 1
INTRODUCTION

A sound mind in a sound body.

How often do we come across this quote?

We have probably been hearing about it since childhood. But have you stopped to ponder on what it means? A sound mind directly affects the well-being of the body. Only when a person is mentally stable can they perform their best and achieve what they want.

We almost always keep a secondary backup for everything. We don't want to lose the things that are important to us and are willing to do anything to preserve them. But why do we not care about the most precious thing we all own?

Why isn't this the case with our health?

God has provided us with the three best things to combat this fear. These things are power, love, and a sound mind. He has also given us the right and will to make specific decisions and take care of our health. It is one of God's most profound blessings. Yet, many of us do not take care of and maintain our health.

Out of everything in this world, the least importance is given to heath, whether physical or mental. It is very easy to get lost in the daily challenges, which deliberately affect our body and mental stability. In today's competitive world, one must remain healthy to succeed. But it is crucial not to overlook our physical, mental, and emotional health. If we have a sound mind, it directly affects the overall quality of our lives will most likely be much better.

The human body and the brain are interconnected. A healthy body goes hand in hand with a healthy mind. Likewise, the brain impacts our thoughts, behaviors, and emotions.

Like the body is prone to illnesses, the human brain can also suffer from diseases and impairment. The only difference is that, unlike physical illnesses, mental health is not awarded with as much attention and acceptance.

The truth is that mental disorders can inflict much more damage than any physical illness if not addressed properly. Unfortunately, even when common mental disorders affect millions of people all around the globe, a very small proportion of the sufferers seek help. Many different conditions are recognized as mental disorders. The main ones being anxiety disorders, mood disorders, psychotic disorders, and food disorders.

Let's briefly discuss them. People suffering from anxiety disorders dread specific situations, respond with fear, and display physical signs of anxiety, panic, and even rapid heartbeat.

A mood disorder, also called an affective disorder, includes prolonged feelings of sadness and even fluctuations between periods of extreme happiness. The most common mood disorders are depression and bipolar disorder. People who have these disorders have extremely inflexible personality traits and experienced unexpected mood swings that are difficult to comprehend.

Eating disorders include extreme personal attitudes and behaviors towards one's diet. The most common eating disorders include obesity, anorexia, and bulimia.

The most destructive of all the mental disorders are psychotic ones that require help as soon as possible. They cause impaired awareness, reasoning and impede thinking. Hallucinations and delusions are the most prevalent symptoms—schizophrenia and dementia are common examples of psychotic disorders.

The extent to which these mental disorders affect people ranges from person to person. They can cause problems at the workplace, schools, or social relationships. They lower a person's self-esteem, creating tension, havoc, uncertainty, and stress in their lives. Long-term unattended mental disorders also induce suicidal thoughts. They also lead to drug and substance abuse.

If these mental disorders are so grave, why are they not addressed that often?

Why is there a stigma attached to mental disorders?

Why do people not share what they feel?

That's because of the stigma associated. Often, when they do reach out, their issues are brushed aside. It's very common for someone to be labeled as dramatic, emotional, or just showcasing attention-seeking behavior when it could be a silent cry for help. In that case, it is easy for the person to feel judged and misunderstood by others. This further isolates them.

There's also the perception that if someone has a mental health issue, they will not function properly. For example, if someone is depressed, they won't be able to smile, or if someone has anxiety, they would be scared of every single thing around them. Stereotypes make it easy for people to dismiss those who don't show atypical symptoms of their mental illness.

But the truth is that high-functioning individuals can suffer from mental health issues and still get the job done. It's not healthy, but they may be just better at masking or hiding what they're suffering from. For example, a person with depression can laugh as happily as someone who doesn't have the same condition. It doesn't mean that they're faking their depression.

There are more than 200 classified mental disorders ranging from the common ones like depression, anxiety, and bipolar disorders to rarer ones like dissociative identity disorder. Even though advancements are constantly being made in the field of medicine, the stigma around mental health disorders means that society repeatedly fails to truly understand them. The impact of such an approach to mental health is nothing less than disastrous.

Until recently, mental illnesses and disorders were taboo topics. Media perception was also not favorable. In popular films, most serial killers, kidnappers, murders, etc., were shown to have mental health problems. People were and still are uncomfortable talking about this subject. Although progress has been made, several misconceptions, stigmas, and prejudice against people are still a problem.

Researchers have helped to break down the stigmas into three types.

The first is public stigma, which involves the pejorative attitudes others tend to have about mental health issues.

The second kind of stigma involves a negative attitude towards oneself, including low self-esteem, self-efficacy, and shame about their condition. For example, a person starts to believe that they are incompetent and useless because of their mental health.

The third kind highlights a more systematic problem. Institutional stigma entails policies that govern private or government institutions and organizations that inhibit the opportunities for betterment for people with mental disorders. People working in such corporations are more likely to get fired based on their behavioral patterns.

Many people suffering from mental health problems find difficulty in talking about it with others. People who suffer from these disorders are usually termed crazy and insane. These further tend to aggravate their conditions, and all in all, they stop sharing what they feel.

There's also shame associated with seeking professional help for mental health issues. More than half the people don't receive help for their conditions. They feel ashamed about their psychiatric disorders because they believe that they are exhibiting symptoms that are generally considered weak and bad by society.

Society and the people around us tend to have a benchmark for what it means to be *normal.* Anyone who fails to live up to the mark is considered dysfunctional. Moreover, having their feelings constantly dismissed and not having concerns taken seriously often isolates people, forcing them to stop talking about their problems.

Denial is also a key concern. Most people who suffer from disorders find it difficult to accept that they need help. To them, the ramifications and backlash of admitting to having a mental illness outweigh the benefits of seeking help.

Some people are simply unaware that what they might be suffering from is a recognized mental health issue. Lack of knowledge and availability is a practical issue in rural areas. These areas usually have fewer medical facilities, and the situation for mental health care is worse there. Rehabilitation services and psychiatric treatments are also very expensive.

Some people cannot afford the treatment or medications prescribed to them. Certain treatments are also not covered by insurance. Moreover, minors are less likely to have insurance and are usually at higher risk. People also avoid going for therapy because they are often scared of the severity of their disorder and the treatment they might receive.

Due to the lack of knowledge and awareness, people think that those suffering from mental disorders are crazy. There is also a common misconception that mental illnesses and disorders are very rare.

People suffering from mental disorders are shunned and are mistreated, and a popular myth is that it makes people non-functional. They also have a perception that people can never recover from mental disorders once developed. While on the other hand, proper treatment may help people overcome their problems almost completely, and they can go back to leading an ever-normal life. The empathy received by a sick person is not shown to someone who is emotionally unwell.

Owing to the various portrayals by media and past techniques, there is a violent image attached to the treatment. Thankfully, the old disturbing conceptions and treatments of shock therapy and padded rooms are mostly void now.

People fail to comprehend that instead of belittling people, the more they support the sufferers, the faster the chances of recovery. They may also face more trouble in their workspaces without comprehensive cooperation.

It is crucial to take ample steps if one is feeling distressed or requires help. Despite the stigma surrounding mental disorders, one should feel free to get treated as soon as possible before the condition worsens. The ugly truth is that in the long run, the only true friend one has is themself. Nobody will actually care about you or take accountability for what you do. Therefore, you have to take a stand for yourself and love yourself.

Sometimes, it gets difficult to identify the disorders and symptoms causing the ailment. But, under no condition should you self-diagnose. To identify the underlying conditions, it is essential to get accurate diagnoses of the problem, which will help in undergoing proper treatment. Furthermore, the more information you have, the more are the chances of successful communication with the therapist.

Psychiatric prescriptions and medications alongside psychotherapy can be an effective mode of treatment. During the therapy, you learn more about your feelings, condition, mood, and behaviors and the coping mechanisms to control the issue.

If not tended to immediately, mental health disorders can take a serious toll on an individual's health. In addition, it might heighten the associated risks, especially if the person suffers from hallucinations or suicidal ideation. For example, without help, a person with social anxiety has a higher chance of becoming anti-social, seriously affecting their quality of life.

Eventually, the person might engage in substance abuse and alcoholism. Hopelessness and insecurity can also lead to death. If you know someone around you who is suffering, help them out or, at the least, get them treated, as it can potentially save the life of a loved one.

Everyone has the right to live and enjoy their lives to the fullest. We should help those around us and encourage them to find courage and fulfillment. We can help them either individually or on a much broader platform. By addressing the stigma surrounding mental disorders, we will help someone and promote awareness society lacks.

Start from your own house. So much of the stigma has to do with family and friends being oblivious of the victim. So the very initial step is to use all the resources available around us and learn. Spreading awareness among people is no hard task today. Social marketing campaigns can be very effective.

The National Alliance on Mental Illness (NAMI) offers various resources on how one can help in reducing the stigma of mental disorders and illnesses. One thing each and everybody can do, even without the aid of social media, is to talk about it as much as they can. Hold public gatherings and seminars and raise awareness as much as possible.

Social media has become a safe space where people consistently speak up about their mental health and care for others. Make the best use of social media and educate others, respond to their misconceptions, and cater to their confusions, especially in rural areas where these problems aren't addressed much. Introduce various programs targeted at vulnerable people, constituting minorities, migrants, and people affected by disasters and conflicts. Introduce mental health awareness seminars and interventions at workplaces. Promote mental health awareness activities in schools.

Also, root for free mental consultations for people who cannot afford therapy or insurance. Reiterate the fact that it is basic human etiquette to help others in need and distress. Compassion surpasses all the feelings, and just as how ill people are treated; mental disorders should also be catered to similarly. Also, encourage equality between physical and mental illnesses. Drawing contrasts between them both and highlights how considering them both is equally important.

All in all, this might help in cooperating with the ones suffering and in bringing courage. It might also boost their confidence and strike out the alienated feeling they might possess. It will help in promoting acceptance and respect and having people see them as an individual and not as someone with sickness can make the biggest difference for struggling people.

Chapter 2
LIFE WITHOUT ILLNESS

Growing up, I had a very healthy and happy life. I did my best in everything and pretty much succeeded in anything I set my mind to. I considered myself as God-gifted because every project or goal I embarked on I would accomplish profoundly. I was always a popular, athletic, and outgoing child who did fairly well in school but never applied myself academically, but when I did, I got great results, and everyone around me was proud. I was always more into playing, sports, and having fun.

I knew my way around everything. I got into high school and was average in my studies. I was always ambitious and hardworking, and at a very young age, I started working as a paperboy, and soon enough, worked at a local grocery store. I recall working on Sundays at the grocery store during my senior year in high school while also getting paid triple times the usual pay per hour. I learned a strong work ethic from my father; he too was a very hard-working person, and I aimed for very high in life.

I met Cheryl, my now ex-wife, at the University of Dayton at the end of my junior year, and I fell in love immediately. I walked up to her at a bar and offered to buy her a drink. She was gorgeous, the kind of person who was very particular about herself, her looks, and also worked on staying fit. She was also very good with studies, and I knew she was good for me.

So when she fell for me, I considered myself the luckiest person on earth. Among the few good things that my life incorporates, Cheryl is the best thing that ever happened to me. We shared many similarities and likings; she also enjoyed sports like me. She is a beautiful woman, full of life, intelligent, caring, and upbeat.

Most importantly, she is the mother of my two beautiful children, Allie and Jack. She chose me out of all the handsome, high-profile guys she was surrounded with, and I was just a beer-drinking frat boy. She made me into a better person, and I spent some amazing times with her.

She was the person I gave my everything to, and I loved her to death. The time we spent together was delightful. We got married in 1986, and the years I spent with her and my children I consider them the golden memories and the time of my life.

My children absolutely loved me. One thing Cheryl and I always taught our children was respect and humility. Allie and Jack respected me a lot. They were really close to me, and they had unconditional love for me.

During the later years of our marriage, after moving to Atlanta, Cheryl got a promotion and was mostly out of town as her job demanded traveling, and I often had the kids to myself. I was working full time at Coca-Cola, traveling an hour each way, and had to drop them off and pick them up from daycare and used to cook for them. Jack was into football, soccer, baseball, and basketball, while Allie was into dance, basketball, soccer, and volleyball. Whenever I was home or got free from work, I would help coach them. We had a lot of fun together.

I helped them in their studies too. When Cheryl would be home, we had fun together, visited places, and went on trips mainly to visit Cheryl's parents in Florida. The children loved playing sports, and we managed our schedules accordingly. After the divorce, I would see the kids every other weekend, one evening during the week for dinner, and never missed their games. The children looked up to me for everything.

I was born into a Catholic religious family, and so was Cheryl. Even before the children were born, we made our regular trips to Sunday Mass.

My wife and I never missed church. We are both Catholic. We were members of the St. Alphonsus Liguori Catholic Church in Zionsville, Indiana. My daughter Allie was baptized there. Jack was baptized at the Holy Cross Catholic Church in Batavia, Illinois. Allie had her first communion in Saint Andrew Catholic Church in Roswell, Georgia. Jack had his first communion in St. Brigid Catholic Church in Johns Creek, Georgia, and both my children had their confirmation there as well.

We inculcated the same teachings into Allie and Jack. Cheryl was stricter on them than me, but we didn't want to impose teaching on our children; we taught them to respect all people. As Allie and Jack grew up, they really looked forward to Sundays and spending time in the Church. After we separated, we still went to church together as a family at St. Brigid, but eventually, Cheryl decided to go back to St. Andrew's without me.

We made sure not to compromise on our children's upbringing. Even after the daily strenuous tasks, Cheryl would come home and spend time with Allie and Jack and pay attention to the children. Our priority was them and their education. We would take turns in helping the kids with their homework.

I worked full-time during the summer while studying in college and did manual labor jobs and paid for tuition with the money I saved up by working and through student loans. I worked for Warner-Lambert for eleven years until 1996, when I joined Coca-Cola.

In 1983, I got my first sales job with Genesee Brewing Company. I sent a letter to the vice president of sales, Jack Genier. He called me in for an interview, and the very first thing he said to me when I sat down before him was that my cover letter was the best cover letter he had ever read in his entire life. He subsequently gave me an entry-level sales job of $21,000 a year and a free brand-new red Ford tempo. I had one old great business writing teacher in the spring of my senior year in college and got an A. I owe a lot of my business success through the years to her.

I started working at Coca-Cola in January of 1996. I was hired in the national accounts at the company, and initially, my job was going well. Owing to my practical and communication skills, I signed up AutoZone for a new beverage agreement with Coca-Cola. The agreement was to put up coke coolers and products in all three thousand plus AutoZone stores nationwide.

It was a very good job, and I was making a decent base salary of about $75,000 a year. Moreover, I also earned a lot of bonuses and was also given stock options. Furthermore, the company also promised me a pension if I served them for a long time.

I was living in Alpharetta during my job at Coca-Cola, and the distance to the company was horrific. Despite all the advantages, the best prospects, better facilities, and coordination, the commute was brutal from Alpharetta to downtown Atlanta to Coca-Cola every day. It took me an hour each way to reach the office, and I abhorred it. My position also demanded wearing a suit daily.

I still remember the stress of commuting to Coca-Cola every day and having to rush home to get the kids from daycare right before it closed, and taking care of the kids at night while Cheryl was traveling, was very hard. It was easier when Cheryl worked from home and would get the kids from daycare, but it was difficult when I had a long commute.

Cheryl also got a promotion with her job, and between my and Cheryl's money before the divorce, we had over one million dollars. We led a very happy and content life. Years later, I got my dream job with SAP in lead generation business development, but not until many years working for poor jobs and horrible bosses. Some of the companies I worked for were GE, Lanier business systems, Point Clear EarthLink, and Eclipse Networks.

Life took an ugly turn when I lost control of my life in the fourth quarter of 1998 when I was diagnosed with schizophrenia. Everything that was meant to be for me just drifted away, and I was left empty-handed. Nothing was in my control anymore. I lost the most important things in life, and everything I dreamt of, for my family and my future, was destroyed. I only wish I could turn back time and fix everything.

I had always been successful in my job, had a beautiful wife, two wonderful kids, and lived in a beautiful huge house in Alpharetta, a nice suburb. I had really achieved everything that I wanted to achieve, and we had a lot of money in the bank. I loved my wife very much. I think, with what I was going through, I had a hard time accepting things and was probably trying to blame her for what was wrong with me.

I got hospitalized twice in 1999, and each hospitalization lasted almost five weeks. They were mainly for medication management, stabilization, and group therapy. Finally, I was cleared to return to work, but on my first day back to the office, I was escorted out of the building by security and was fired from Coca-Cola in August of 1999.

One month later, Cheryl filed for divorce. As a result, I had to leave the house and find an apartment to live in. I remember residing at a hotel for three days while I searched for a place to stay. Eventually, I rented a two-bedroom apartment. During my first few nights in the apartment, I slept on the floor with only pillows and bedding. My struggles were endless. The clinical definition of a sexless marriage is sex ten times or less per year. After my daughter, Allie, was born, I noticed my wife didn't want to have sex with me—not nearly as often as before. She even didn't want to kiss me anymore. I wasn't man enough to address it early on. I was afraid to confront her about it. As a result, when we would go extended weeks without sex, I sought physical female affection elsewhere—not an affair just sex. I think Cheryl was just not into me anymore. When I look back, our marriage became more like a business partnership, and I think Cheryl was always in competition with me. I never suspected she was having an affair until we moved to Georgia, and I got sick with a mental illness. I just thought she didn't enjoy sex anymore. To be honest, maybe she just didn't enjoy having sex with me anymore. After years of reflection, I think she just didn't love me anymore or even question if she ever really did. After I got ill and attended multiple group therapy sessions, I got feedback from multiple people who said, "You need to take back some control." I told Cheryl that I wanted to take control of the finances. I had always given my salary and bonuses to her, and she paid the bills. Her response to me was "over my dead body." Soon thereafter, she filed for divorce.

A true story I want to share with you. We were recently married, and I was promoted and transferred to Indianapolis from Pittsburgh. Cheryl had to leave a job she loved and started working at Merchant's Bank in Indianapolis as a system analyst. She didn't like her new job. We rented a small one-bed one-bath apartment for a few months while our brand new three-bed two-and-a-half-bath house was being built. One Saturday morning, it was cold and snowing outside, and

SCHIZOPHRENIA

Cheryl was angry with me. I left the apartment to take out the garbage quickly, without a jacket, to the dumpster. When I returned to the apartment, Cheryl had locked me out. I had to beg her for fifteen minutes, asking her to let me in. As I was outside the door, pleading with her, in the cold and snow, it was at that moment I questioned whether I made the right decision of getting married.

Cheryl divorced me because I started to act irrational and paranoid. In addition, I became very rude towards her since she wasn't spending much time with me, and I accused her of being a lesbian. We weren't sleeping together, and I suspected that she was having an affair with a man she said she had met on an airplane. I noticed that they knew each other when they met at my daughter's recital because they smiled and acknowledged each other. When I confronted her, she admitted meeting him on an airplane. However, I still didn't believe her.

Since she handled all the finances in our marriage, I also suspected she was stealing money from the marriage by shopping for clothes and returning the items, stashing away the money.

My suspicions turned into delusions which made it impossible for her to live with me. Truthfully, I didn't want a divorce, and I still loved her. I only wished we had more intimacy in our marriage. Her priorities were the kids, her job, and then me if I got lucky. She traveled all week because of her work, while I was also working and watching the kids.

Then she would come home on the weekends, ignore my needs, and play tennis on Saturdays and Sundays, all day with women in the neighborhood. For some reason, she was drifting far from me. Before my illness, I remember while driving home from mass one Sunday, Cheryl yelled at me as I drove and asked for a divorce. At another instance, after she got promoted and started earning more money than me, she said to me, "I don't need you anymore."

This devastated me, and I told her that I didn't want her to need me; I wanted her to want me. Finally, we separated in 1999, and the divorce was finalized in 2001.

Chapter 3
Diagnoses

When I started to feel paranoid, Cheryl knew there was something wrong with me. I was reluctant to admit to it. I didn't think there was anything wrong with me. But I had hurt the people around me terribly without realizing that I needed help.

Eventually, on Cheryl's insistence, I went with her to my first mental health appointment. The doctor was very certain that I was displaying symptoms of schizophrenia. You know, when a doctor tells you that you have a mental illness and you might have to take medicines for the rest of your life, that is a tough thing to swallow.

I had a tough time accepting my illness. It felt like just a moment ago, everything was perfect in my world. Then, suddenly, I started feeling I was ripped off of the control I had on my life. My world was unraveling.

I knew that nothing was ever going to be normal again. I didn't know who to trust. I missed the specific part of my life where I worried less and lived happily with my kids and wife around with their love and support.

Much to my dismay, I was hospitalized at Ridgeview Institute multiple times and at Charter Peachford once. Each of those hospitalizations lasted for five weeks, and they were mainly for medicine management stabilization and group therapy. Now that I look back, it was helpful; they both were great places for me. I was hospitalized the final time at Ridgeview Institute in 2002 and then again for a year at Georgia Regional Hospital in 2017 and 2018, when my condition aggravated.

SCHIZOPHRENIA

In August 1999, I was discharged from Ridgeview Institute and went home. After that, if not all, I did feel much better and peaceful. However, when I went to work, I was escorted out of the building by the security from Coca-Cola off the premises. To this day, I don't really know why I was fired. However, I knew I had started to feel isolated at work.

A month after losing my job, Cheryl filed for divorce, and I had to leave my house. After that, I reflected on where I had gone wrong. One Saturday morning living in Alpharetta, I came downstairs in the kitchen. This is before I was diagnosed with a mental illness. Cheryl was in her robe, standing in the kitchen. I gave her a hug from behind and kissed her on the side of her neck saying, "Good morning. I love you." She turned around and pushed me away and said, "Get off of me." I was just trying to show love and affection. I was really hurt by that reaction, but once again, I did nothing. Marriage vows say you stay together for richer or poorer, in sickness and in health all the days of your life. The reality was we were in a sexless marriage. I got sick and lost my job because of it. I surmise she didn't love me because if she did, we could have fixed everything together. My wife already told me a year earlier "I want a divorce" and "I don't need you anymore" after she started making more money than me. I now believe my illness and losing my job was her ticket to get full physical custody of the kids and child support. And that is what she got.

It was all ravaged.

I didn't know what to do.

I was also very angry at that time. I didn't have much to live with. I had no job or income source; I only had $401k money in my account. I didn't even have furniture or utensils, neither much food nor clothes too. Eventually, I negotiated to get some furniture from my ex-wife as part of the assets we were splitting between us and was able to get all my clothes.

She did agree to it, but I was alarmed when she asked for a police presence at the house when I had the movers come and take the furniture and my clothes. She was threatened with my presence. I was on medication and was still able to see my children. Unfortunately, the medicine I was on was not working well for me at that time.

Maybe she was fearful of me and for the kids. But I never physically hurt her or my children.

It led me to believe that taking medicine was useless and so was seeking therapy. I don't blame my wife for getting a divorce; I do understand that I was reckless and that she didn't want to live with a person who wasn't acknowledging the gravity of their illness and wreaking persistent havoc in their lives.

After being hospitalized twice in 1999, I was hospitalized for inpatient and outpatient three more times until 2002. That is when I met Dr. Arun Munjal, a psychiatrist at Ridgeview Institute. He was asked to see me by another doctor for second opinion. Back then, the FDA had just released a new drug, Geodon, and he prescribed me that. Geodon worked like magic for me. It turned someone completely psychotic, like myself, into a normal person or how I sometimes think of myself—I went from being possessed by the devil to a normal law-abiding, loving, and productive Christian citizen.

Even though I was not working at the peak of my illness, my ex asked the divorce judge to set child support. Because I was making $75K annually prior to being fired, he set my child support, at $1,350 monthly, assuming I could still afford it and find a job at that income level.

We shared legal custody of my two children, and my wife had primary physical custody. My daughter, Allie, was eleven, and my son, Jack, was six at the time. Therefore, even though the child support was based on my base salary of $75K per year and even though I had lost the job, it was assumed that I would earn in the same salary bracket.

But I never got back to that level of income until 2013, after my support ended. After several years of paying Cheryl $1,350 per month, I told her that I could only afford $1,000 per month since I was making $45K per year only. I didn't even have enough money to hire an attorney and go back to court to get it reduced. So I decided to talk to her, and she agreed. So I paid child support for twelve years from 1999 until 2012, and the total amount I paid exceeded $200K.

Prior to one of my hospitalizations, after the divorce, I wasn't working. I couldn't work due to my instability and impulsive behavior. I was having a hard time finding a job. At the same time, I was paying rent and child support from my 401k money. Even though I was paying child support, my ex-wife wouldn't let me see the kids because I said I was off my medicine. I told her I was fine and posed no threat to any of them.

She wanted me to take my medications on time and properly, so she took me to court to assure that I was taking medicine before seeing the kids. I had to get a blood test monthly for a year with an out-of-pocket cost of $150 for each test to prove that I had Geodon in my system, and the results were sent to my doctor and Cheryl.

At one point, I remember that I got very frustrated and stopped my treatments. This happened before I met Dr. Munjal and was taking Geodon. My brother and dad tried to convince me, but I did not budge. Finally, when words failed, they both came to my apartment to try and force me into getting treatment. I wasn't letting them inside when they came to the door, but they weren't taking no for an answer and pushed their way into my apartment.

To save myself from the unwarranted attack, as I believed it to be, I jumped out of the second-floor window to get away from them as fast as I could. Soon enough, the cops arrived, and I was picked up and sent to Ridgeview Institute for treatment again. Also, since my family had me arrested, I spent three days in the Alpharetta jail.

When I was off the medicine, I got unrealistic thoughts and became very paranoid. I thought everyone was out to get me and harm me, but the side effects of the medicine were weight gain and sexual impotence. In addition, I was gaining weight rapidly and slowly inching towards obesity, which came with many other problems as well.

After my ex-wife and I divorced, we shared legal custody of our two children, with her as the primary custodian. I had visitation rights. My visitation was every other weekend and one weeknight during the week, and we alternated holidays.

My kids were very athletic, and I got to see them all the time, a lot during the whole week. Cheryl used to call, asking me to pick them up from practice and take them to school. We had an excellent working relationship co-parenting the kids, and I'm very grateful to her for allowing that to happen. After our divorce, I would consider

Cheryl, my ex-wife, as one of my very close friends. I did then and still, today, have a tremendous amount of respect for her.

I lived in an apartment for three years until I finally bought my house in 2003. When I had visitation with the kids, and before Allie moved away and went to college, even when she was older, she still came over to my house every other weekend with Jack.

"Allie, you're all grown-up now. You don't have to come over on the weekends anymore if you don't want to," I said.

She replied, "Dad, I like coming over."

I said, "Okay, sounds good."

Allie used to ask me about dinner when she was with me on the weekends during their visitations. She always required me to make a good meal for the three of us herself, Jack, and me. In a way, I was grateful to her for pushing me to be a good dad and learn to cook better for the three of us. When Allie went away to college, Jack still came over every other weekend.

However, my ex-wife Cheryl was traveling an awful lot for work. And when she was out of town, Jack would stay with me. While Jack was in high school, he was living with me over 60 percent of the time. I was still paying $1,000 a month for child support to my ex-wife. Though Jack lived with me most of the time, I never stopped giving Cheryl child support even when I wasn't as financially well off as she was.

I remember being arrested for trespassing at my ex-wife's house because I was off my medicine and went to pick up the kids on my normal day of visitation. This was before I met Dr. Munjal. She knew I wasn't taking medicines and called the cops.

When I was brought to the Fulton County Jail psych unit, I waited with the other inmates to talk to the judge in court. I saw attorney Tom Ford, as I was leaving the court. I asked him for his business card while I was handcuffed, and he gave it to me. I contacted him from jail. I told him the money I possessed at that time totaled $571K, in my 401k retirement account. He didn't believe me and shrugged me off.

Later, my parents came to Atlanta to help me; they talked to Tom Ford and convinced him on my behalf, and thanks to Tom, I was released from jail, and my parents paid him $5,000 to represent me. I am very thankful to God for my parents, who stood by me through thick and thin and pulled me out from every trouble.

I was a grown man who had money in my account, but I had no job, and I didn't know what to do. And I knew that nobody would hire me knowing my condition. So I was full-blown, once again psychotic, off my medicine, and displayed unpredictable behavior.

Tom Ford was a good attorney, and he knew that all I needed was hospitalization, therapy, and medication management, which is exactly what he negotiated for with Fulton County. So I was incarcerated for five days at Fulton County jail, and I was taken directly from the jail to the Ridgeview Institute by my mother and father. I didn't even have any probation whatsoever. So I went back on the medicine in 2002 until I went off it one time in 2015 and was back on it in September 2017 and continue it 'till this day.

My biggest regret after going off the medicine this final time is losing my relationship with Allie, Jack, Cheryl, and my sister Betsy. I used to be very close with my children and talked to them often in person and via phone. When Allie came back home from college after graduating and working in the Atlanta area, I used to see her for dinner twice a month.

I enjoyed getting together with her and having a beautiful father-daughter bond. Unfortunately, the last time I met her for dinner was in 2015, when I was off my medicine and acting very irrationally. Once, at dinner, I asked her.

"Is Peter hitting on you?"

For some reason, I thought Peter, her mom's boyfriend, was trying to hit on my daughter because he asked me on the phone when he and Cheryl broke up, to have Allie call him. I told him I wouldn't do it, and regardless of any evidence, I thought he was hitting on Allie. He even told me he practically raised them, Allie and Jack. That made me very angry. In one instance, Jack even shared with me that he didn't like Peter.

I made Allie very upset. She started to cry and subsequently left dinner by herself. She was in her early twenties at that time and a working college graduate. I felt awful. The illness was causing me to lose everything that I cherished.

I used to have a wonderful relationship with my sister Betsy. She would call me on her ride home from work almost every day, just checking up on me after my diagnosis. Of course, by then, I would already be home and tired, but I enjoyed those conversations. She called me a few times a week, and we would just talk for thirty minutes or so on the phone as she drove home.

It was great to stay connected and talk about things in our personal lives, and I considered her not only my sister but a good friend. She helped me when I went off my medicine in 2015 and when some bad things started happening to me. Especially in 2016, before I was arrested, she was bringing me food on the weekends. She pleaded with me to get back on my medicine, and I told her nothing was wrong with me.

I was adamant. Physically, I was feeling so good while off the medicine, but mentally, I was not doing myself any favors. She got so frustrated with me that she stopped bringing me food because I was so uncooperative. I was and still am sincerely apologetic for my behavior towards her and my family because I didn't listen to them.

I got enraged whenever the topic was brought up. It wasn't because they weren't trying; it was me being too bullheaded, believing there was nothing wrong with me. Even though I was feeling so good physically but mentally, I was not there.

A week before my son's graduation from college, I didn't have a job anymore and didn't have a car. I contacted Jack through text and asked him about his graduation. He told me not to bother coming to his ceremony, even though I didn't have the means to drive to Birmingham and Samford University. I was devasted and broke down. I never expected Jack to drift away from me as we had a great relationship. We talked and shared everything with each other.

While off the medicine in 2015, I was driving home from work, and I was manic. I didn't even recognize that I was speeding in a school zone, and there was a school bus that had stopped on our street in the neighborhood. I drove around it, not even realizing that I had broken the law. A woman in the neighborhood witnessed the scene and complained about me.

I received a letter and complaint from the Forsyth County Police Department. I'm so glad and thankful to God that I didn't end up hitting a child getting off the school bus.

Earlier, when I first went to Ridgeview Institute during my hospitalizations, I was intimidated by the doctors and afraid about the procedures. So I threatened to run away.

I remember my mom pleading with me; she reminded me how the treatment was important for my family and me. She constantly reminded me of my kids.

"You will never see them unless you get treated," she told me. So she finally convinced me to do it. Because if I didn't, I would be sent back to jail.

In 2015, when I was off my medicine but still working and less psychotic, I bought a new garbage disposal and had it installed by a Russian plumber I found on Craigslist. Then in 2016, when the madness found its way back to me, I removed the garbage disposal and returned it to Lowe's when I needed money for food. That is how distorted my thinking became.

I even made up a weird conspiracy in my mind. The Russian who had installed my garbage disposal mentioned that my sink plumbing was put in incorrectly, so I had the urge to remove it. So I removed the kitchen sink and threw it in the garage because I always wanted a new sink even though I didn't have the money to get one.

I was completely isolated. My children weren't talking to me; my sister, who also lived in the Atlanta area, was not talking to me either. I had run out of money, electricity, and eventually gas. My sister Betsy was paying my water bill, but I had no access to hot water. Hence I took cold showers and drank from the faucet.

My condition deteriorated with isolation, and I started to remove the hardwood floor in the front hall. Since there was a small gap showing, I stuck the end of the crowbar there and completely tore up the floor. I started wasting the money I already had on useless, pointless things like painting the kitchen wall even though it was perfectly fine.

I painted the kitchen and family room but couldn't finish because I ran out of money and didn't have enough to buy all the paint needed. I took apart the ice machine in the refrigerator. I thought it was faulty because I had found two small screws missing. I considered it a scam and a conspiracy to get to me because it was made in China.

I would go on the back patio to lift weights. I was down to about 219 pounds from about 245 pounds in January 2015. I felt so good physically, but mentally I was paranoid and thought everyone was against me. I started to believe that my neighbor was coming into my house and moving things.

He and his wife were a nice young couple, but for some reason, I targeted him as the person who was coming into my house, and it was a false psychotic belief. I even called the cops once and told them that someone had broken into the house. The cop came and informed me that there was an unlocked window in the family room that was probably letting burglars into the house.

In 2015, before I lost my job, I went to a new psychiatrist for a few appointments because she had advertised that she helped patients get off antipsychotic medicine. She tried to prescribe medicine, but I refused. She even asked for a joint appointment with my grown daughter to convince me to go on my medicine.

My daughter came to the appointment and tried to convince me, but I turned it down. At the end of the appointment, I asked her for a hug, like we usually did while parting ways, but she refused. I was heartbroken.

Off the medicine, in 2015, before I lost my job with SAP, I even ordered new furniture. I spent over $5,500 on new furniture for the family room and moved the old furniture into the living room. My old furniture, which was in the living room, was given to me by Tom, my brother. I was also angry at him for some reason.

Just because of that, I threw it out by the road. I was making poor decisions by spending money when I didn't need to and also because I was manic and flying high and making good money at the time at SAP.

It all came to an end when I lost my job on 21 October 2015. I'm sure everyone in SAP couldn't understand what was happening with me. In fact I was a top performer, the number one performer in North America from my group, and suddenly, everything went spiraling out of control.

After SAP fired me, they sent me a letter warning me never to contact any employee at the office, and if I did, they would take legal action. The truth was I had become irrational, unpredictable, and paranoid. I was afraid of myself; I wouldn't go to work even. So SAP had no choice but to fire me, even though the job could be done very easily remotely working from home.

On the way back home from the office while working for Coca-Cola, and when I didn't have to pick the kids from daycare, I would occasionally stop at a strip joint for a drink. It was there that I got introduced to cigarettes. My smoking habit escalated after my divorce.

Before I bought my house, while living in an apartment, I smoked a pack a day. Later after I bought my house and on weekends when I didn't have the kids or any games to watch, I would go to a strip club at noon on Saturday and smoke cigarettes and drink wine all afternoon before I would come home around dinnertime. That all ended in 2007 after my DUI arrest. I haven't had a cigarette since.

In 2015, I remember how angry I would get towards my brother Tom and my ex-wife, Cheryl. I sent her a petty text message once, telling her to feel free to change her name back to her maiden name. After that, I started to think the same things that I had once thought years earlier that she was having an affair behind my back while we were married. I also assumed she was stealing money from the marriage because she planned to leave me and get child support. I even questioned if she ever really loved me, and I wrote all of my assumptions down in the annulment information that I filled with the Catholic Church when I was off my medicine.

Tom came to my house and rang the doorbell when he was in town. I was so angry, I glared at him and almost threateningly asked him what he wanted. I didn't even let him inside the house. Now that I reflect on it, I realize how awful I had been. He didn't do anything to me; he always meant good for me.

I just had anger towards him because he and Dad had me arrested and thrown to jail the first time; they forced me to get back on medicine. It was that grudge I held against my brother. Early in my illness, I remember I even questioned my dad, asking him if he was actually my father. Despite his answers, I remained unconvinced, and I even asked him if I could see his driver's license.

He knew I was not sane and let me look at his license, but he still did not disown me. Instead, both he and my mom stuck with me and knew that it was just the illness that made me act that way.

Schizophrenia is a serious mental disorder in which people interpret reality abnormally. It may result in hallucinations, delusions, extremely distorted thinking, and behavior that impairs the daily functions of a person. It can be disabling and seriously affect the quality of one's life. Additionally, not all forms of schizophrenia are the same. The one I have is schizoaffective disorder. It is schizophrenia with mania.

After the divorce, I always struggled to find the right well-paying job since I lost my job at coke. It wasn't until 2013 that I found the right and good-paying job at SAP. I loved my job at SAP and was very good at it. I had two female managers that were great. They encouraged me to perform constantly and challenged me with extra work, but I welcomed it because it provided more opportunities to make bonus money.

My base salary was only $50K per year, but I was killing it in bonuses. I was doing this while on my medicine until I went off in January 2015 and then lost my job at SAP in October 2015. I used to get contacted by many people on LinkedIn for other opportunities. Unfortunately, after I lost my job at SAP and got in a car accident in November of that same year, I could not capitalize on the companies that contacted me on LinkedIn.

I was out of my mind and couldn't even focus on finding a new job. All I could think about were things around me directly. If I could have just focused on going back on my medication and taking advantage of my experience at SAP, I would have had many better job opportunities.

Chapter 4
TROUBLES WITH LAW ENFORCEMENT

In 2002, while being hospitalized at Ridgeview Institute, Dr. Munjal told me, "If you don't take this medicine every day as I prescribe it, you will end up in either dead or in jail."

He was right. Getting off the medicine was the worst decision I have made to date. However, it would take hitting rock bottom through a series of unfortunate yet, avoidable events for me to come to that realization.

When I was off my medicine in 2001, it was my weekend for visitation, and my ex-wife, Cheryl, knew I was off my medicine. I went over to her house to get the kids, and she refused to open the door. I saw my son, Jack, through the side lights of the front door. He was excited to see me, but Cheryl asked me to leave, and so I did.

She, later on, called the cops, and I was arrested for criminal trespassing. I spent five days in jail while the judge ordered me to get admitted at Ridgeview institute as part of a plea deal, and the charges were dropped.

In 2003 I bought my house for $223,000 and put $70,000 down. I wanted my kids to have space in a yard whenever they would visit me. I used my $401k money for a down payment. I was also paying $1,500 a month in rent for a three-bedroom, and my mortgage payment was only $1,060.

In 2007, I got a DUI after spending the afternoon at a strip club when I was only trying to have some female interaction. I was on probation for one year, and I was on my medicine. I would do that once in a while, but after my DUI, basically, I stopped going to strip clubs.

I was on Geodon from 2002 until 2015 and went off my medicine in January 2015. Dr. Arun Munjal was my psychiatrist, and he prescribed my medicine monthly. While off my medicine, I took my kids Jack and Allie to a family wedding in Rochester, New York, in July of 2015. I'm not sure if they noticed or my family noticed, but I was going paranoid.

I was involved in a minor car accident in November of 2015 when the car in front of me stopped to make a right-hand turn. It was moving at 45 mph. It was 9:30 a.m., and I wanted to change the time on my clock, so I looked away.

When I looked back up, I slid into the back of the SUV ahead of me, which I had failed to notice had stopped. Thankfully, no one was hurt. Later on, the cop gave me a ticket for failure to stop.

A few months later, I was walking by and thought to check the CCTV footage. I stopped by a bank next to the entrance of the parking lot where the accident took place.

"Do you have a security camera that might have gotten the accident video?" I asked them.

"We don't," they said.

I left the bank and walked to another bank where I had an account. I didn't believe what they had said to me. I went back to the bank, BB&T, the entrance to where the accident took place, and this time, I asked to speak to the manager and asked for the footage again. They again denied having any video.

I left, and they called the Johns Creek cops on me. I was picked up by the cops outside the bank in the parking lot. At first, I was surprised.

"What's the reason for my arrest?" I asked them.

"The bank complained about you and called 911." They informed me. "Can we have your ID?"

I refused to produce it, which ultimately resulted in six cops showing up. I was still not cooperative, so they wrestled me against the trunk of a car, and I was arrested and taken to jail. After that arrest, I spent five days in the Alpharetta jail and then transferred for forty days to Lumpkin County Jail. During this entire time, I didn't even know what I was being arrested for.

At the Johns Creek Courtroom

When I showed up in court, walking in a suit for the disorderly conduct charge in Johns Creek, my sister Betsy was in court with attorney Tom Ford, who had previously helped me with my DUI charge in 2007.

"I'll represent myself," I told the judge.

I was paranoid and declined to have Tom Ford represent me. That was a terrible decision.

When the prosecutor refused to meet with me in the back of the courtroom, I complained. The judge asked the cops to get me, and six cops tackled me to the ground, face down on my stomach and with my hands behind my back. I was kicked in the stomach by one of the cops and in the ribs by another. I was arrested and taken to Alpharetta jail then transferred to Lumpkin County jail for forty days.

A good public defender Mr. Rodgers got me out of jail, and I was given one-year probation in Fulton County. When I was given the probation, the attorney told me, "You don't have to appear for the probation, but I strongly warn you against performing or getting involved with any other misconduct for a year."

That was the only way to save me from probation.

My brother and sister, Michael and Betsy, picked me up and took me to a doctor immediately following that incarceration at Lumpkin County jail. But, I refused treatment after speaking to the psychiatrist for an hour; I was furious. I even refused to take a ride to my house with my brother and sister and decided to walk home by myself.

At that time, I was living with no money, no car, no job, and I didn't even have any electricity or gas in my house, but I was still convinced that I didn't need medicine or treatment, and I was doing just fine. Little did I know my life was going to get even worse.

When I went home, I started thinking and believing that people were coming into my house whenever I left it. It made my paranoia and distrust of people worse. I didn't trust anyone.

Another time in 2016, I was walking on McGinnis ferry road not too far from my home. After getting food, I was walking home from a restaurant and had my wallet, watches, and the engagement ring that I bought for Sameitria in a backpack.

The ring was worth about $1,000.

I also had my laptop, and I would usually go to Target or McDonald's that were within two miles each from my house, to use their Internet.

As I was walking home on a sidewalk, a cop pulled over, stopped me, and started questioning me.

"Where are you going?" He asked. "Why do you have a backpack?"

I couldn't understand why he was interrogating me like this.

"Why are you asking me those questions?" I asked him. "I am not breaking the law. I am just walking to my house after working on my laptop."

"I'm gonna need your ID," he told me, and I gave it to him.

"Can I look in your backpack?" He asked, and I complied. However, once he saw the diamond ring, he looked at me suspiciously as if I had committed a crime.

"Whose ring is it?" he asked. "Have you stolen it from someone?"

I immediately became defensive. "It's mine. People have been breaking into my home when I am not there, and because of that, I have to carry it with me."

He was skeptical, but eventually, he let me go, but not before another cop showed up. That's how unreasonable the cops are in Forsyth County. I was shocked. I had done absolutely nothing wrong, and out of nowhere, the cop stopped me and started questioning me.

People who are mentally ill need help, care, and love. Even the tiniest of harsh situations can flip the world for them. Jail is not the place to be while you're mentally ill. I was constantly getting in trouble while I was in jail because of my paranoia and discomfort there.

Oddly, jails have rules of conduct there too. Someone who is constantly disrupting things or wreaking havoc in there is put into lockdown. That means that you can never leave your cell under any circumstances. You're not allowed any privileges. There is no free time in the open-air cell to get fresh air. You can't watch TV, nor play cards or other board games with the other inmates.

At one point in time, while I was in the medical unit at Forsyth County jail, I was on lockdown, and I spent three months in my cell without ever leaving. I had a shower and a toilet, but all my food was being brought to me. I couldn't go anywhere, and this all happened after an original charge of misdemeanor.

While I was at Forsyth County jail, they even lost my paperwork after the judge ordered me to be evaluated at Georgia Regional Hospital. So I spent three more months in there, longer than I had to. Locked in my cell, I couldn't go anywhere and got mentally worse by the day. I was getting into trouble everywhere I turned.

While in jail, food is the king. Everybody fights for it. It is because the nutritional value is pretty low, and the quantity served is not enough to satiate a grown-up. So you look for any way to get more food; you have to figure out a way to do it or slowly starve. I went into jail, weighing 219 pounds, but I had lost weight drastically by the time I left; after exactly one year, I was down to 158 pounds.

One time, while in jail, I was walking handcuffed in line with other inmates, and the guard suddenly issued a command.

"Stop and face the wall!"

That's because a woman was coming on the other side of the hallway. I didn't stop fast enough, and the guard hit me on the back of the head with his forearm, and my head smashed against the wall. That is how you are treated in jail. Some guards are nice, most of them are really mean.

By December of 2016, I was in the medical unit of Forsyth County Jail and had been incarcerated for several months and held without bail with no trial date set for my misdemeanor. I had a single room with a separate shower and toilet and a bunk. Thankfully, I had no roommates.

I got in trouble with the jail staff for hoarding too many books in my room. I mainly read the Bible and many incoming monthly volumes of old Catholic Magnificat books. For some reason, I don't even know why I was placed in lockdown in a padded cell in the medical unit. After being in that cell overnight, I was let out to use a bathroom in the morning. As I was walking towards the bathroom, the guard was behind me yelled at me, "This is my house! You do what I say! This is my house!"

I felt my rage boil over in a split second, and I was so angry at him that I tried to hit him in the face, but I missed. Immediately, I was wrestled and tackled to the ground by three guards. I was placed in a restraining device, in which I could not move my hands, arms, and legs, and I could barely see or breathe. They kept me in this device for several hours, and all I could do was lie on the floor of the padded cell.

The only way you could urinate in this padded cell was through a drain in the middle of the floor. But I had to ask to use a toilet for a bowel movement; it was the only way to get out of the cell. After this incident, I picked up my felony charge the very next day.

The day after Christmas in 2016, I was transferred to the SummitRidge Hospital in Gwinnett County. It was like a country club compared to jail. I was there to be evaluated. But since I was feeling so good physically, I refused to take medicine, again. I thought there was nothing wrong with me, and everyone else was in the wrong.

I ate as much food as I wanted. I was being served three meals without any restrictions. Finally, after a week of being there and going through the group sessions, I was still off the medicine. However, they said I was having too much fun and wasn't taking this seriously. So they transferred me back to jail.

In retrospect, if I had accepted their medical treatment and started taking medicine while I was there, I might have been able to save my house through the help of family and could have avoided more suffering.

While I was at the SummitRidge Hospital, my sister Betsy was kind enough to bring me some clothes. I looked and felt great in the new clothes. Next, I called and successfully asked a tax accountant to visit me at SummitRidge.

"If you do my taxes," I told him, "I will pay you from the refund of the taxes of my 2015 filing."

I also told him about my current condition, that I was at SummitRidge.

"Can you contact my mortgage provider to save my house from being foreclosed on?" I asked him.

He agreed to meet me, and we spent over thirty minutes together. Through the interview, I was determined, but I was also convinced that he wasn't a good fit because of my paranoia.

I should have just been happy that he agreed to come to see me and help me. But for some reason, because of my illness, I thought he had bad intentions towards me with no proof whatsoever. That is how bad I was when my paranoia would get a hold of me.

But I knew I had to pay my mortgage. I was trying to help myself well, but I couldn't get out of my own way. I questioned everybody about everything they were trying to do for me. Even when they followed my instructions, I tried to analyze and overanalyze everything, turning the positive into something negative.

I was constantly making up false reasons for why people were mistreating me. I always thought that I was the victim because of the actions of others around me when, in reality, I was the one doing everything to myself.

I even had people tell me that I was very intelligent when in reality, I was psychotic. My former public defender, Joseph Stauffer, told me that.

"You're very intelligent," he'd say, even when I was so mean to him, yelled at him, and passed rude comments on his physique and weight, all while he was trying to defend me.

When I was brought into jail, I was paranoid and was given an ID by the jail staff. An ID is required to have any phone service in the jail. I was afraid to give my ID to the guard as I changed clothes. When I refused to provide him with the ID, they tackled me naked to the ground. All because I refused to give him the ID that I was holding in my hand.

In February 2015, my daughter took me to the Forsyth County court and asked the judge to tell me never to contact her again. I had sent her a voicemail at 5:00 a.m. after Super Bowl Sunday and drove to her house, my ex-wife's house. I rang the neighbors' doorbell to see if she was still living there because she wasn't responding to my calls.

I was convinced that something horrible had happened to her and was devastated.

The final event was in the summer of 2016, after I was released from the Lumpkin County jail. I was back in my house, not paying my mortgage. I had no electricity or gas, and my mother was paying my water bills. Then, one day, I was on the back patio and saw my neighbor walking into his garage.

I started yelling at him because I thought he was coming into my house without permission. As I walked towards his garage, in his front yard, he warned me, "Get off my property before I call the cops."

I immediately turned around, and as I was leaving his yard, I yelled at him, "If I ever catch you in my house, I will kill you!"

Then I went inside my house and went to bed. Soon enough, a female officer came to my door, but I refused to answer it. After viewing her from an upstairs window, I think the same female cop that pulled me over years earlier thinking I didn't have a seatbelt on.

About a month later, I was arrested outside a Home Depot while taking back tools to get some money to buy food. Six cops arrested me. The charges were misdemeanor, trespassing, and terroristic threats.

I spent thirty days in Forsyth County jail and then the judge let me out on my recognizance as I was awaiting trial and told me to contact probation. When I was released from jail, I walked back home from Forsyth County Courthouse and jail.

It was a ten-mile walk.

I didn't have a working cell phone anymore and tried only once to call the probation officer from an AT&T cell phone store but couldn't reach anyone.

Five days later, in September of 2016, I was arrested again at home as I was cutting my grass with no shirt on. I was taken to the Forsyth County jail and spent the next year in Forsyth County jail.

I picked up additional felony charges in December of 2016 for trying to punch a guard in Forsyth County jail. Because of my misdemeanor charges and the charge for assault on a correctional officer, I was granted no bail.

I waited in Forsyth County jail until September of 2017, that is when I went to the Georgia Regional Hospital. It wasn't until that time that I started to take medication again. I was released from the Georgia Regional Hospital in September of 2018.

When I was released, I went back to Forsyth County jail for a few nights because I was due to appear in front of the judge for my felony conviction. I was given five-year probation, no jail time, and one hundred twenty hours of community service. I was given a light sentence because I was a first-time offender for a felony which was a blessing. In November of 2018, I received a year of probation for the misdemeanor charges from Forsyth County.

When I was given my felony conviction and probation, I went to New York with my brother Tom who came to help me, and while I lived there, we shared the expenses until May of 2020. I went back to court in November of 2020 and asked the judge to terminate my probation.

He agreed, and I hired an attorney, Joseph Stauffer, my original public defender. He was so nice and only charged me $500 for the motion.

While in jail in July of 2017, my sister Betsy along with my older brother Michael took me to court to get guardianship and conservatorship over me. The thought was that they could force me to get back on my medicine and take over my financial affairs.

My monthly mortgage of $1,060 had not been paid for a year. My sister and my ex-wife, Cheryl, and my daughter, Allie, testified against me, and my rights were taken away from me in July 2017. In June of 2017, my house was auctioned off, unbeknownst to me, while I was in jail.

After my sister got guardianship and conservatorships over me in July of 2017, she was notified by a police officer that she had to get all of my things out of my house immediately because the house was going to be taken over. Thankfully Betsy had put most of my furniture and clothes into a pod and into storage.

I am very grateful to her for that. Ideally, I wish my family would have paid my mortgage instead of paying for an attorney to get guardianship and conservatorships over me. That is my biggest regret from this whole ordeal, losing my house and the relationship with my children.

My house was auctioned off for $267,000, and my mortgage was $154,000. As of August of 2021, I finally received the remaining balance of my equity, which was $89,624.88.

When my son, Jack, was a freshman in college, I was stable on my medicine; my ex-wife, Cheryl, asked me, as always, if I could drive Jack back to school. It's a three-hour trip each way to Birmingham. I am always early whenever I have to be somewhere, and Cheryl knew this. She said to me, "Please don't be early and wait in the driveway." I don't know why that would make her angry; I was usually twenty to fifteen minutes early by habit. I was out running errands, and it was Sunday early afternoon. I had about thirty minutes to kill and, therefore, decided to pass the time at Newtown Park about a half mile from my wife's neighborhood and house. I backed up my car in a parking spot so I could see everything with a view and was listening to the Braves game. As I was parked, a very young John's Creek police officer drove by and stared at me. I don't like cops, don't trust them, and think most of them are egotistical bullies. After he starred at me and against my wife's wishes, I decided to leave and parked in her driveway about fifteen minutes early. That cop followed me approached me and got out of his car. He asked if I lived there and asked for my ID. I was enraged. I said, "Why? What did I do wrong?" I told him what I was there to do and would not give him my ID. I told him you are harassing me, and I did nothing wrong. He said he was suspicious of me because the way I was parked, assuming I was purposely concealing my license plate. He finally left and said to me, "I know who you are," after viewing my plate. One of many examples of why I distrust cops.

Another instance was in 2007. I was stable on my medication, and on a Friday night, I had an attractive slim black escort named Hazel visit me at my home. We had drinks and made love, and it was a fun night of female companionship and intimacy. The next morning, I left the house early around 8:00 a.m., driving a mile from home going to the grocery store. A masculine female cop pulled me over and asked for my license and registration. I complied and waited in the car. She eventually came back with my documents and said she thought I wasn't wearing a seat belt. Why, to this day, do I think I was targeted?

In 2016, I went to Stein Mart, one of my favorite stores, and I went there to give back a suit I had purchased in early 2015. Because I didn't have the receipt, Stein Mart refused to take it back. I was angry as I couldn't believe the store manager wouldn't take it back after all the business I had given them over the years. The store manager knew I was angry, and as I left the store, she called the cops, and I was banned from going back to that store in the future.

When I was out of money and food, I used to go to the Sprouts Farmers Market in Johns Creek to get free samples of bulk nuts. I would often go two miles each way from my house just to get some food. Once, I walked ten miles each way to the North Fulton community charities, where they had a food bank. I worked there for my community service after my DUI arrest. So that is how I knew they had a food pantry.

They turned me away because I had a Forsyth County address.

While I was still paranoid, after having a couple of drinks at a bar, I stopped at St. Brigid Chapel to pray. While there, I disturbed other people who were praying because I said, "God is not always listening."

I was asked to leave by the people in the chapel. So I immediately left.

And on my way home on a two-lane side of the road, I failed to pull forward next to a police officer. I'm terrified of police officers. I did nothing wrong. I didn't break the law; I just didn't want to pull alongside the police officers, so I didn't pull my car all the way forward.

I wasn't drunk because enough time had elapsed since I had my two drinks. The cop followed me and pulled me over. I was petrified.

"Leave the vehicle," the cop asked me, and I refused. He tried to pull me out of the vehicle, and I still refused. So they gave me a ticket. I don't know what the ticket was for, but they gave it to me. Later when I went to Johns Creek court to pay the traffic ticket, my church complained to Johns Creek police about me, and the judge ordered me to stay out of St. Brigid and Johns Creek for a year. I couldn't believe my beloved St. Brigid called the cops on me.

After I was taken into custody at Johns Creek court, my ribs were killing me after being kicked by the cops. So they took me to Johns Creek hospital. But I decided not to get an x-ray because they didn't tell me how much it would cost.

I was mentally ill, and they then took me to Alpharetta jail for five days and then transferred me to Lumpkin County jail for forty days. My cell phone was stolen at Alpharetta jail, it never made it to Lumpkin county jail and was never returned to me. When being admitted to Lumpkin County jail, I was frisked by the guard. He purposely ripped down my back pocket, tearing my suit pants.

In 2016, before I went to jail, I got hit twice by cars pulling out of a parking lot while I was walking on a sidewalk and crosswalk, and a third time, I was walking on the side of a forty-mile-per-hour road, McGinnis ferry Road. I got clipped in the arm while walking with an umbrella, and I was thrown ten feet. I was off my medicine but got no severe injuries, just really sore bones, and also, the car didn't stop.

Whether in jail or a hospital, being incarcerated is the worst thing you can ever imagine. While at Georgia Regional, I got punched in the face twice, once by a young twenty-year-old black man. He gave me a black eye that lasted a month. I got hit another time by a white man in his thirties. He punched me in the chin, but there was no real damage.

The black young kid punched me because I complained that he was using the community phone well past his fifteen minutes allotted time. The man in his thirties punched me because I think he didn't like me. He wasn't at the hospital long. They sent him back to jail quickly.

I believe consistently receiving the sacraments of confession and communion helped me through my illness and incarceration in jail and at Georgia Regional Hospital.

SCHIZOPHRENIA

While in jail in 2016, I was punched in the mouth and received a clean cut on my lower lip, where my lip meets my cheek, and I got eight stitches there. It was from a young kid who was a real problem and constantly got into fights with everybody. He took medicine every day because I watched him go to get his medicine in the morning.

I was put into a new cellblock and was trying to use the phone. Every time I used the phone, they yelled from their cell so I couldn't hear, and I told them to shut up.

The next day when they opened up the cell, everyone came out into the common area. He and another kid came at me, and both of them punched me. One hit me with a razor blade. I remember how embarrassed I was to be paraded through the emergency room in my jail outfit to get stitches at the local hospital in Forsyth County. All the people in the hospital were looking at me, and I must have looked really gruesome.

I remember the nurse who did the stitches for me and a police officer who watched over the whole process were really nice. The nurse was very attractive, and she evidently wasn't scared of me. She also made me feel better and told me that there wouldn't be a bad scar.

A number of weeks later, when it was time to get the stitches out, they took me out to a private practice doctor's office near the jail in Forsyth County. I remember sitting in the waiting room with the police officer who was with me, and I was still handcuffed. I just remember the people waiting there looking at me like, "Oh my God, there's a guy from jail in our waiting room."

"You'll have a scar," the doctor said as he removed my stitches, which I do, but it is not that noticeable.

After I was released from jail in 2017, I was sent to Georgia Regional Hospital in September 2018. Then I was sent back to jail for three days while I waited for the hearing for my felony charge. After my felony charge was determined, I was released from jail.

Thank God my brother Tom was there to pick me up. He was very nice to me and let me stay with him until I decided what I was going to do. My sister had full guardianship and conservatorships over me. She was furious because I hired an attorney at Georgia Regional Hospital to defend me on the misdemeanor charges.

That attorney was Tom Ford, the same one who had represented me in my DUI case back in 2007. For some reason, she did not like Tom Ford, and she wasn't happy that I didn't consult her when I made that decision, even though I did not ask her for any money to pay for Tom Ford.

I borrowed $5,000 from my brother Tom. Because my sister was making it so difficult to get money from her and I didn't know where I was going to stay, my brother offered for me to go back to New York with him and stay with him. We could split the rent while I decided what I was going to do.

My credit was in shambles, and my sister had all of my money. I got a lump-sum payment of over $35,000 for disability, but my sister limited my access to it. She only gave me like $600 or $700 at a time. She had my furniture and clothes in storage.

Before I went to New York, I got some clothes from storage, but I still needed to get all my clothes and things once I found out where I was going to stay.

I asked for approval from Forsyth County to transfer my probation from the felony charge to Ontario County, New York, and they agreed. My probation officer in Ontario County, New York, was Karen Grout.

Karen was really nice. I saw her every month until I left New York to return to Georgia in May of 2020. I did not have to pay any court costs or any fines for my felony probation. That was a blessing. While on my felony probation, I did my one hundred and twenty hours of community service at the Habitat for Humanity Restore in Canandaigua, New York. I lived in a one-bedroom apartment with my brother for about one and one-half months until we were able to secure, in the same complex, a two-bedroom apartment with one bath.

While in New York, I had to get a new bank account. I had $600, and I went to the Chase Bank in Perinton, New York, to set up a new one.

I told him I was on Social Security Disability, but I did not tell him my sister had guardianship and conservatorship over me. Through the grace of God, he said, "I can change your Social Security direct deposit to go to your new account."

So we did that without approval from my sister.

The next month, in October 2018, I started receiving direct deposits from Social Security to my account.

My sister was a little angry with me.

"How were you able to do that?" She asked. I was worried that she would try to change it, but she never did. It made it so much easier and gave me a bit of independence. I had some money, and I could manage my life with it. I paid half of my rent and utilities responsibly and started saving money.

While in New York, I was saving an average of $800–$900 a month. I used that money to pay off some debt I had incurred after being in jail and Georgia Regional Hospital and hire an attorney to get my guardianship and conservatorships reversed.

In December of 2019, I hired an attorney in Forsyth County, Georgia, Mandy Moyer, while I was in New York. She specialized in probate law and was happy to take my case. I paid her $3,250. It was a reasonable price for an initial payment compared to other lawyers asking me for $10,000. I had done some research and found out that the only thing I needed to do to get my guardianship and conservatorships back was to find two approved doctors who could say that I was fine and no longer needed a guardian or conservator.

However, after further consultation, Mandy Moyer used to work for the probate judge who was overseeing the case. My sister's attorney filed a motion and complained to the judge. She said she did not want that to happen. So as a result, Mandy Moyer removed herself from the case. And gave me a partial refund.

I am grateful to Mandy for giving me a template of how to file a motion to do the work on my own to get my guardianship and conservatorship terminated. With the help of some government stimulus checks and saving money while living with my brother, I moved back to Georgia in May of 2020.

I had a total of $12,000 in savings. I had sold my furniture to my brother and only had my clothes. I checked in at the Extended Stay America hotel in Alpharetta, Georgia, three miles from my old church, St. Brigid, and three miles from where my ex-wife and children live. I haven't seen my ex-wife or children since I've been back in Georgia, but it's good to be back here with the good weather, and I was able to take care of the things I needed to get my life together.

After settling, the one thing I had to focus on was getting my guardianship and conservatorship back. I couldn't do anything about my felony probation because my lawyer told me we could petition the court to get that terminated after two years, so I had some time to wait on that. Now I had a template to file a motion on my own with the Forsyth County probate court with the same judge that terminated my guardianship and conservatorship rights and gave them to my sister and funded by my brother.

I had the hardest time finding an approved doctor that would take my case to evaluate me and fill out an affidavit on my behalf saying that I no longer needed a guardian or conservator. However, I finally found a psychologist in Dacula, Georgia, who took my insurance. Her name was Shirley Boone Sanford, PhD.

An assistant, Brandy Valasquez, conducted the psychological testing, and it took four and one-half hours. It was 100 percent approved and paid for by my insurance, which was a blessing. I was also able to get an affidavit from Dr. Munjal, who I had seen for years and was back seeing him when I came back to Georgia. He agreed that I no longer needed a guardian or conservator, but wanted to evaluate me for six months.

He assured me that I could manage my own affairs since I was stable enough and back on my medicine of 180 mg of Geodon every day. Even though my sister had guardianship and conservatorships over me, she still retained an attorney who was working on her behalf to charge me for attorney fees.

I had sent my sister text messages saying she no longer needed an attorney, but she never responded. She was not communicating with me freely. When I moved back to New York, it took me almost two months to convince my sister to give me money so I could buy a car.

I wasn't sure how much I would pay for a car, but I wanted to pay for a car in cash, so I didn't have a car payment, especially since my credit was awful. She was trying to tell me what kind of car to buy and how much money to spend, and I just told her I was looking for a decent car. So I was going to spend around $20,000.

She thought the amount was too much. At the same time, I convinced her to send me the $20,000 anyway. I ended up buying a 2016 Ford Escape, which was 7000 miles for $18,600. I still have that car, and it has 27,700 miles currently, and it's paid for.

I did that while on the medicine. Then, after being in New York for about six weeks, right when we were about to move into a two-bedroom apartment, I had my furniture and clothes from storage move from Georgia to New York. I put the furniture in my mom and dad's garage and my spare clothes in her basement.

When my brother and I moved into the two-bedroom apartment, I furnished the place as my brother did not have any furniture. It was so nice to have my full wardrobe of clothes again after living in jail in Georgia Regional Hospital for two years not having my own clothes.

It is the little things that you take for granted that you miss when you're deprived. For example, I continually asked my sister Betsy to send me the rest of my lump sum payment from Social Security, but she didn't send me the rest until I came back to Georgia after May 2020. I used that money to pay off the remaining debts.

Using the medical evaluation from Dr. Shirley Boone Sanford and Dr. Arun Munjal, my psychiatrist, I filed a motion to get my guardianship and conservatorship terminated from Forsyth County probate court in September 2020. Unfortunately, the judge refused my petition because he said I filled out the paperwork incorrectly.

In his judgment, he said I needed an additional doctor to petition the court, and he would still use the evaluation from Dr. Shirley Boone Sanford and Dr. Arun Munjal.

According to Georgia law, you can use a psychologist, a psychiatrist, a regular medical doctor, or even a licensed clinical social worker as proof to get guardianship and conservatorship back. With that in mind, I decided to go back to my former therapist Constance Cromartie, who is a licensed professional counselor. The probate court asked me who would do the third and final evaluation, and I had to submit Constance Cromartie as that person so they could send her the paperwork.

The court rejected Constance as an evaluator because she was just a licensed professional counselor and not a licensed clinical social worker. It was at that time I had to find another doctor. I asked Constance if she could recommend a licensed clinical social worker that could help me out. I was having the hardest time finding somebody to do another evaluation of me for the court. Most doctors did not want to put their name and reputation on the line on my behalf, in fear that something bad would happen to me again because of my illness.

Constance recommended that I go to Stephanie Robbins right here in Alpharetta, Georgia. Stephanie agreed to take my case and agreed to see me for six appointments, at $150 per appointment. She did not take my insurance. She said she would agree to see me but could not guarantee that her assistance would help in the termination of my guardianship and conservatorships. She had to see me first. After six appointments with Stephanie, she agreed and filed with the court and filled out the paperwork to terminate my guardianship and conservatorship.

At this time, the previous Forsyth County probate judge unexpectedly retired due to sexual harassment allegations, and his replacement was the former public defender, Daisy Weeks, who represented me in the original guardianship and conservatorship trial. Because of this, the case was sent over to the Georgia Superior Court judge, the same judge who handled my felony conviction and probation and who terminated my felony probation in November of 2020.

Judge Bagley then heard the final case and asked Mandy Moyer, my former attorney, to represent me. Using my three affidavits containing the various doctors' recommendations, Mandy came to the final hearing and asked Stephanie Robbins to attend and testify on my behalf. Judge Bagley ruled that my guardianship and conservatorships be terminated immediately.

I also learned at that hearing that the interpleader case handling the proceeds from my house auction was also at his court, and if I needed to get that money, I would have to file a motion to that court to get those funds released.

An interpleader case is when there are monies that multiple people are trying to get access to. Then the attorney representing the company that did my mortgage auction files the interpleader case, so the judge could decide who would get the money and what amount of it. Most of those people seeking funds from my house auction equity had already been paid by me to restore my credit.

The only two people they needed to be paid is Forsyth County probate court for $9,600 for Daisy Weeks who represented me in the original proceeding for guardianship and conservatorship and is now the probate court judge and a little over $3,400 from my sister Betsy's attorney who handled the case in the guardianship and conservatorship. It wasn't being paid anymore by Betsy and my brother Mike, and they wanted it to be paid by me.

In an attempt for speed and simplicity, I contacted both attorneys for probate court and my sister's guardianship and conservatorship attorneys. I agreed to pay what they were asking to the court, and the probate court attorney agreed to file a joint motion on all of our behalf to have them be paid and the remaining balance to be given to me.

On 4 August 2021, Judge Jeffrey Bagley awarded me the remaining balance of the interpleader case from my house equity in the auction of $89,624.88. I owe a debt of gratitude to Judge Bagley since he gave me a favorable sentence of five-year probation on my felony charge. After two years on my felony charge, he terminated my probation and gave me my guardianship and conservatorship back.

After I had overwhelming evidence that it was no longer needed, he awarded me the remaining balance of my house proceeds for the interpleader case, and I put all this behind me since I moved back to Georgia in May of 2020. As further testament to handling my affairs, I made all of these court motions, all the doctor's appointments, all the research, all the communication, all of it while on my medicine fully stable and under the care of Dr. Munjal.

I should never have been held in jail for an entire year without bail while waiting to get evaluated at Georgia Regional Hospital. It wasn't until I got to Georgia Regional Hospital that I could get back on my medicine, get stabilized, and move on with my life.

Even though I was offered medicine while in jail, I needed a medical environment to get stable and be with a doctor in an environment that I could trust. I had no trust in the doctor that came to the jail once every two weeks.

Chapter 5
SINS AND FORLORN

Throughout my life, I struggled with the seven deadly sins: lust, gluttony, greed, sloth, wrath, envy, and pride. At times today, I still struggle with lust, gluttony, and greed, but there is always room to change, and I try my best to keep them in check. I have my greed as a motivating factor for me to write this book.

I lived a sinful, adulterous life, something I am not proud of, and I seek God's forgiveness. I think that He punished me for it with my mental illness. Even twenty years after my divorce, I still feel guilty daily, even after going to confession multiple times for cheating on my wife before the divorce.

I was very sexually active, and performing in bed, and having sex was always very important to me. Unfortunately, I wasn't a faithful husband. When Cheryl would be busy or out of town, and we would go extended weeks without sex, I went to massage parlors to have sex and felt awfully guilty afterward. I often used to justify my infidelity on the reason that my ex-wife wouldn't make love to me consistently. I craved her love and attention, especially after the children were born, and I now know how wrong I was.

In retrospect, as I look back on it, she probably didn't want to or had probably lost interest in me. She didn't want to be intimate with a gluttonous and lazy husband. But of all the women I have been intimate with, I never forgot how lovely Cheryl was. Even after the divorce, I missed her.

I had a serious intimate relationship with a woman named Jackie. The sex was great, but I knew that I didn't want to marry her, so I never introduced her to the kids. She lived in the North Georgia Mountains, and I would visit her every other weekend to spend time with her when I didn't have the kids for visitation.

As I grew older, the only way I could perform sexually was by taking Viagra or Levitra that Dr. Munjal would prescribe for me.

There was another pretty African American escort that I saw three times, Hazel. I met her after my divorce. I wasn't with her for a long period, but she was a very nice and beautiful woman. I got a bit more serious and limited hooking up with random women after that.

I used to go to the library occasionally to work. I had met Sameitria in the library ten years earlier when she was in her late twenties and was twenty years younger than me. My laptop was broken, and I went to the library to check my email.

She came and sat next to me on another computer workstation. I couldn't believe how cute she was. I also had no idea how old she was. I introduced myself when I was leaving and asked her if she would like to get coffee or lunch sometime in the spur of the moment. She smiled and asked for my number, which I gladly gave her, and two weeks later she called me.

We casually dated on and off for over ten years. Our relationship became intimate, and I fell in love with her and eventually asked her to marry me. To my dismay, she returned the ring three days later.

"I'm not ready for marriage," she told me. "I will be more than happy if we just keep doing what we were doing."

I was shattered; I really wanted to marry her.

Nevertheless, I loved her a lot and didn't want to lose her, so that's what we did. The ring I bought for Sam was a fat engagement ring. Ironically both this ring and my college class ring and my watches were in my house when it was auctioned off. When my sister picked up my furniture and things, my jewelry never made it out.

God knows where they are now.

When I was in jail, I never lost my faith in God and the Catholic Church. I called my parish priest, Father Tri, at St. Brigid Catholic Church, and he came twice to jail to give me the Holy Eucharist and hear my confession. Ironically, it was Father Tri who motivated me to make a change in my life.

SCHIZOPHRENIA

Before going off my medicine in early 2015, during a confession, I opened up to him entirely about how lonely I was and how I had no wife, had no support, and was overweight. I told him about my illness, infidelity, and my desire to be remarried in the Catholic Church with my current girlfriend, Sam.

It was that conversation with him when he shared some amazing insight with me.

"Your illness is, in fact, the devil preying on your life," he told me. I agreed with him but to an extent. I had assumed that it was because of my weight that my girlfriend, Sam, wouldn't marry me, and if I lost some, I'd have a better chance of convincing her to be my wife. We used to go out to eat often, and many times she would come over to my house, and I would grill out and make dinner, and we would drink wine together. It was so much fun. I loved her and her company.

While I was in jail, Sameitria (Sam) came to visit me on two different occasions. She made me really happy whenever she visited me, and I actually waited for her. I wished my kids would have come to see me, too, but I guess they didn't know how to handle the situation. I don't think anybody in my family was communicating with my children about my situation.

By this time, my children had fully grown up; my son was graduating from college, and my daughter was already a college graduate. They could make their own decisions. My sister Betsy came to visit me in jail a few times, and my brother Tom also came to visit me. Tom was living in New York at that time but came to Atlanta for some skin cancer treatments, and while he was in Atlanta, he came to see me.

Only video visitation was allowed when my brother and sister came to the jail to see me for visitation. We always ended up getting in an argument as I was very difficult to deal with. I was angry and confused because I was having a hard time in jail while trying to figure out why nobody was helping me and why nothing was being done to get me out.

I wasn't communicating with my lawyers, and I had no bail options. I would talk to my parents via phone from jail, and they didn't know what to do. I was very psychotic. My mind was constantly racing from one thought to the next. I constantly thought somebody was out to get me, from the jail personnel to the doctor in the jail to even my family members.

I didn't trust anybody. However, I felt comfortable and loved by Sam, my girlfriend, and by my parents. The support that came from Father Tri from the church also helped somewhat calm me.

So after that confession and meeting with my primary care, Dr. Sunjatha, I decided to go off my medicine to lose weight. I filed for an annulment in the tribunal of the Archdiocese of Atlanta in the spring of 2015 while I was off my medicine. My annulment was granted one and one-half years later.

When I was at Georgia Regional Hospital, after being in jail for a year, I got back on the medicine and was becoming stable. I called my parish again, asking for communion and confession. Father Neil, the pastor of our parish of St. Brigid Catholic Church, came to visit me once at Georgia Regional Hospital. He sent Father Bill and a Eucharistic minister, who visited a few times.

I even called the prison ministry at the Archdiocese of Atlanta, and they sent a priest that came to visit me twice. He was a very eccentric priest but also entertaining. He was obviously flamboyantly gay, and he was a nice guy. They sent a eucharistic minister as well to give me communion several times.

Finally, as recommended, I called the Catholic Church that was close to the Georgia Regional Hospital, Saint Peter and Paul. They sent a very nice deacon, Tony King, who was an African-American man. Tony came to visit me weekly until I was released. He was also very nice and selfless. I read the Bible daily and prayed for my release throughout my time in jail for one year and at the Georgia Regional Hospital for another year. I would say the rosary, often using my fingers as I was not allowed to have one in jail or at Georgia Regional.

My relationship with my daughter got so bad that she took me to court in February of 2016. She wanted the court to tell me not to contact her anymore. I seriously believe she was afraid of me. I didn't hurt her in any way; I just wanted to talk to her. What possibly triggered her fear was probably the event where I had visited her at her place of work before I lost my job. And then I went to my ex-wife's house where she still lived and tried to talk to her. She wanted it all to stop, so she took me to court. She testified that I was following her in the car in court, but that was incorrect. I never did so.

I went to the courtroom, and my son Jack was there as my daughter Allie testified in front of the judge and brought a recording of about 5:00 a.m. voice message that I sent her after the Super Bowl.

The judge decided in her favor and granted her wishes. I was told not to have any contact with my daughter and that I shouldn't even try. I was devastated. During weekends when I had the kids on visitation, when they were younger, I never missed taking them to church. I truly loved going to mass with Allie and Jack.

I was afraid to go to mass by myself after the divorce for the longest time. But eventually, I overcame that and started going to church not only with my kids but every Sunday by myself at 7:30 a.m. mass at St. Brigid Catholic Church.

I had cashed the 401k money I had from SAP. That is what I used to live for a few months.

I now know there was so much more to the relationship than just intimacy. It has taken me nearly sixty years to figure this out. For the longest time, I blamed my ex-wife for divorcing me when I got ill. I thought she abandoned me. I now realize that it was my own fault that the marriage failed. It was my guilt from infidelity that ruined my marriage and not just my mental illness.

I truly am sorry to my ex-wife Cheryl, my daughter Allie and my son Jack for inadvertently subjecting them to the trauma of a divorce and a broken family, all because of my weak self-esteem and lustful sins. I try now to live a simple life full of kindness and generosity towards all people.

Chapter 6
MEMORIES

I remember before I was officially diagnosed with schizophrenia, Jack was five years old. My wife, Cheryl, signed him up for baseball, and I agreed to be the coach. I played varsity baseball while in high school and so was pretty good at it. Even though it was a very stressful time working at Coca-Cola, commuting an hour each way in heavy Atlanta traffic, coming back home every day, and trying to have practices and games with these young boys, I managed and made some good memories with the kids.

Once, I remember a young single mom came to the first practice with her son, and her son wasn't wearing his glove.

"Where is his glove?" I asked her.

"I didn't know what kind of glove to get him," she replied.

"Is he right-handed or left-handed?" I inquired.

She didn't know that either, and I knew I had to figure it out myself. So I threw a ball to the boy.

"Throw it to me," I told him, and I noticed that he threw it back with his right hand.

"Get him a left-handed glove," I told the mother. And she smiled and was very thankful.

My daughter Allie, as well as my son Jack, were both great athletes. My daughter played volleyball and basketball in high school but eventually focused only on volleyball. Her team was so good that they won the state championship in her senior year. She was selected as an all-state all-star. It was so much fun watching her play.

She also played club volleyball, which my ex-wife, Cheryl, paid for. Allie ended up getting a scholarship at Marist College in New York for volleyball. It was her junior year, and I had never been able to afford to go to New York and see her play volleyball in college.

After I spent years watching her play volleyball in high school, I felt awful about it because I didn't have enough money to travel. In addition, I was still paying my ex-wife $1,000 a month in child support, as well as a mortgage on my house and living expenses. Also, I wasn't making a lot of money.

I finally did manage to get the money to travel and see her during her junior year, Labor Day weekend. I got the money by filing an insurance claim to repair my roof. I paid for the trip along with some frequent flyer miles. I was also able to pay for the hotel room and buy my daughter a TV and some groceries while I visited her.

It was a great trip. Just me and my daughter Allie, and I was very happy. I was proud and glad when I watched her play volleyball for Marist College. Marist College is in Poughkeepsie, New York, and it is not an easy place to get into. I was proud and glad when I watched her play.

My son Jack was also an outstanding athlete. He played soccer, baseball, basketball, and football. Growing up, I think baseball was his favorite sport. But he was never able to make it to the team in high school. He was an awesome centerfielder; he could run and catch so well and was also a decent hitter. I used to play catch with him outside at the house all the time.

My children and I used to play Home Run Derby in the backyard. We would get a bucket of water and dunk baseball-sized pool toys in the water and hit them with a Wiffle ball bat. We had so much fun playing that game. And we also played offense-defense football in the front yard.

I was usually the quarterback, and it was my daughter against my son. We did this on many fall weekends. When my son played baseball, I used to be the scorekeeper for his games many times. I also was asked to be the third base coach many times. When my son, Jack, was in sixth grade, Cheryl, my ex-wife, signed him up for spring baseball. He loved playing baseball, and I thoroughly enjoyed going to his games. I had been stable taking my medication for years. They were social events to me. You get out of the house in the fresh air and sun and converse and chat with other parents. Jack was a great center fielder and even pitched a little. He threw left-handedly but batted right-handedly. Cheryl called me and said she got a call from Jack's school, Holy Redeemer, and said he was missing assignments. Just not even turning in some work and as a result, she is forbidding him from playing baseball. I am a firm believer that everyone makes mistakes and occasionally challenge authority to see what you can get away with, especially young boys. I told Cheryl, "Let me talk to him, but let's give him a second chance." I told her, "We'll warn him that one more missed assignment for the rest of his duration in school, he would not be able to play sports." Jack valued playing sports more than anything. So that is what I did. I told him, "I went to bat for you with your mom. You're getting a second chance. Don't squander this opportunity. No more missed assignments or your sports playing career is over. Don't let me down."

He said, "Thanks, Dad. I won't."

As a result, I never heard Cheryl complain about Jack missing school work ever again. And I got to keep going to watch him play games.

Jack played on an all-star team in baseball. He started playing football in seventh grade at Marist High School in Atlanta. I started watching high school football games at Marist when my daughter Allie was a freshman. I used to go to the games every Friday night in the fall, home and away, until Jack was a senior and graduated.

It was just great entertainment. I was so proud to eventually see my son Jack good enough to play on the varsity. Unfortunately when Jack made the varsity team as a junior in high school, he only played as a wide receiver. But he didn't start; I couldn't understand why he never played on defense.

I asked him why he wasn't getting any reps in practice on defense. He said he wasn't sure. So my son never got any defensive reps in practice and subsequently in the games on defense. By the time my son was a senior, he had really grown up. He was a late bloomer like I was.

Always small and going through puberty later in high school. By the time he was a senior, he was six feet one inch and one hundred and ninety pounds. He also ran a 4.50-yard dash. When it was the second game of his senior year, they played against the number one team in their class, Tucker High School.

They finally inserted him into the starting lineup at cornerback against Tucker. Jack ended up being the player of the game and led the team in tackles his very first start. I was so happy and proud of him. I couldn't understand why he was never getting those reps as a junior.

When he got his playing time as a senior, he made the most of it. To this day, I think if he was able to get playing time as a junior, he would have gotten a full-ride football scholarship. During Jack's senior year at one game, a man who I never knew came up to me and asked, "Is your son number 14?"

"Yes," I replied

"He's a helluva football player," he continued with a smile.

"Thank you!" I replied and was so proud of Jack.

By the end of the year, in his senior year and the end-of-season banquet, Jack was the leading tackler on the entire team as a cornerback. But unfortunately, he didn't win any awards.

I used to be so happy on Friday nights after my son's games that he would come and spend the weekend at my house. My daughter was away at college, and it was just Jack and me. I enjoyed his company. And we used to watch sports together. I always offered to cook him breakfast in the morning. I would go to his room around 11:30 a.m. or 12:00 p.m. and ask him if he would "wake up and join the human race" and have some food.

But he always asked for a couple of McDonald's McGriddles. I thought that he didn't like my cooking for a long time and hoped he wouldn't say anything about it, and he never complained.

I paid money to have a video made on my son's football highlights to be distributed to colleges. I did so because a recruiter had contacted me. He saw Jack's performance on one of his fellow teammates' tapes. The recruiter told me that he knew colleges interested in tall defensive backs.

He ended up being selected by Sanford College in Birmingham, Alabama. Jack did decide to go to Sanford and play football, but only as a preferred walk-on, and no scholarship money. He played for two years at Sanford and started on special teams. But never got in on defense as they moved him from safety, which they recruited him as, to an outside linebacker.

He was now close to six feet two inches and weighed about two hundred and twelve pounds. It was the beginning of his sophomore year, and my son was very athletic and looked very good on the football field.

During this one game, he got a concussion on a kickoff. I was in the stands, and I was petrified. Jack laid there unconscious, and they brought a straight board on the field and transported him to an ambulance.

When Jack was being put into the ambulance, I didn't know what to do. All I could do was just yell out to him because I knew he could hear me. I consoled him and told him not to worry and that everything would be okay.

"Jack, it's Dad. Don't worry. Everything will be alright. I love you."

That was all I could say to him. So I followed the ambulance in which my wife was with Jack as they took him to the hospital. I was terrified at that moment and losing it, thinking my Jack, God forbid, might get paralyzed for life.

He was diagnosed with a concussion and, thankfully, had no neck or spinal injury whatsoever. He just got hit hard and got knocked out. It was a terrible concussion, but he managed to play for the remainder of the season.

I think he was a little tentative moving forward since they weren't giving him any scholarship money. He decided that he wanted to stop playing football after this horrendous event. So he called me in told me that he was afraid to leave football as he didn't want to disappoint me.

We had a father-son talk.

"It is entirely your decision and your life," I told him. "I love watching you play, but you shouldn't push or force yourself for me if you don't want to. Do whatever you feel like doing."

He, along with his mom, decided it was best, since he had a concussion already, to stop playing football. I never missed any of Jack's high school football games and attended almost all his college football games. I tried to make it to all my children's games while in high school and many of their games while they both were in college.

While I was on my medicine, I never had any symptoms. I was overweight, but I enjoyed the entertainment, and I was so proud of them. I used to see my ex-wife at almost all the games. She would have her boyfriend, Peter, with her. I was just happy that she was happy and finally found somebody in her life. I asked my girlfriend Sam to come to some games with me, but she never wanted to.

In 2015, when I was off my medicine, I went to a bar that I had seldom gone to before in Dunwoody. That bar was near my children's high school. Ironically while I was having a glass of wine, Coach Chadwick, my son's high school football coach, walked into the bar and sat, talking to a couple of gentlemen.

When I got up to leave after one glass of wine, I walked over to Coach Chadwick to introduce myself and asked him something.

"Why didn't you let Jack play on defense during his junior year?" I confronted him.

He only told me one thing, "Not everybody is perfect."

Coach Chadwick is the winningest coach in Georgia high school history. I was off my medicine, and this is just one example of how confrontational I was and thought everybody had something against the people I love or me.

My daughter Allie is now thirty-three, and my son Jack is now twenty-eight. Both are former NCAA student-athletes and now college grads and working. My ex-wife Cheryl and I spent a lot of money sending them to private Catholic schools for grade school and high school.

After we separated, my daughter went to public schools for four years, but then they opened a new Catholic school, Holy Redeemer, a half a mile from my ex-wife's house.

"I'll see if we can get the kids in Holy Redeemer," I told her. Jack was entering kindergarten, and Allie was entering the fifth grade at that time. Allie was accepted, and Jack was put on the waitlist. I talked to the principal and insisted that she take both of my children in as I wanted them to go to the same school.

She called me back an hour later and informed me that they had both been accepted. My happiness knew no bounds. It was actually a very good school.

Six months after attending Holy Redeemer, my daughter Allie, while with me for weekend visitation, said to me out of the blue, "Dad, thanks for sending me to Holy Redeemer. I really like it there."

I made that decision while taking medicine I thought since we were divorcing, the Catholic education would be good for the kids. I had a Catholic education my whole life.

When my son was in seventh grade, I was unemployed and was switching between jobs. I was on my medicine and overweight but was still paying my child support.

One day, my ex-wife, Cheryl, called me.

"What are you doing?" she asked.

"Looking for a job," I told her.

"I signed Jack up for flag football at the Newtown Park league," she informed me. "They needed coaches, and so I signed you up too."

I coached my son and daughter in sports back then, and they were very young. But these were seventh- and eighth-grade boys, old enough to give you grief. I was worried. We had about five practices before our first game. In practice, we had to decide the positions to assign players. Everyone wanted to be the quarterback and running back. So I told all the boys.

"The fastest person on the team would be the quarterback, and the second-fastest person will be the running back."

We had a fifty-yard sprint. I told my son in front of all the other boys, "If you want to be a quarterback, you must win the race."

My son won, and he was selected as a quarterback. There was another Jewish boy who came in second and was selected as the running back. It was an eight-game season, and we had one practice a week on Wednesdays and games on Saturdays.

We had our first game, and we lost. Then I decided to get more serious. I asked another kid's dad to help me and be my defensive coordinator. He agreed, and I made up a wristband for my son with scripted plays on it, and we practiced.

I would signal in the number, and he would call the play in the huddle. We were succeeding. We were having success running the ball, but all the boys wanted to try a pass. So we put in a play, a fake running back dive up the middle, and it was a play-action pass and then went deep to that same running backup and the middle for a pass.

I finally agreed with the boys to try it in the game. We ran the play. To my amazement, my son faked to the running back, and then twenty-five yards downfield, Jack hit the same running back he faked to perfectly in stride for a seventy-yard touchdown pass. Ultimately after losing the first game, we finished the season with seven wins and one loss.

By winning the remainder of all the games due to the athleticism and commitment of the boys, we won the flag Football League. It was one of the best bonding experiences I ever had with my son, and I have my ex-wife Cheryl to thank for it.

Another time, when my daughter was studying at Marist High School, she had a research paper. It was Sunday, and she was working on my desktop in my office on the first floor of my house. She was complaining about how much work she had, and she was stressing about her paper. I had an excellent creative writing teacher in high school, Mr. Fay, and another excellent, very old business writing teacher in my senior year at the University of Dayton.

So I was very comfortable with writing.

I helped my daughter with her paper, and by the end of the week, she called me saying that she had gotten an A-plus on her paper, and she was all excited. The phone call made me very happy, and I felt glad that somehow, I managed to help her and make her happy.

I went to a family wedding for my nephew in Charlotte with my children. Jack was playing football and in college and Allie was graduated working in Atlanta. While at dinner and having drinks, Allie was sitting next to me. She turned to me and said, "Dad, you're a good-looking man, but if you lost weight, you'd be a really good-looking man." I was flattered and motivated and knew my daughter loved me when she said that. Another time while Allie was at college, she knew I had a huge stomach and drank multiple diet sodas per day. She emailed me a New England journal of medicine article that said diet sodas contribute to belly weight gain. I immediately stopped drinking diet sodas. I felt really loved by her.

The following letter was written to me by my son Jack the summer before he left to go to college and play football. "Dad, As I sit here and write this I can't help but think about all the things you have done for me. You have been the best Dad I could ever ask for. In spite of all the difficulties you've had you still do whatever you can for me. Big or small they all mean a lot to me. From attending every single one of my sporting events, to those days when you would pick me up from Marist, to coming to help me when I hit a tree. You have always been there. I'm going to miss you next year. I know lately I haven't talked to you much and I'm sorry. I don't have much more time left in Atlanta and I want to make the most of it. I have always dreaded all the times I have to come over and do lawn work, but I shouldn't. I need to be more appreciative. I want to make our relationship stronger. I would love for me and you to go out to eat regularly and catch up on life, football and girls. As my father, I have always looked up to you and felt a stronger connection with you. At times this connection is lost because I don't see you often, but that has been my fault and I want to make sure that doesn't happen anymore. Next year we won't have many moments with me leaving for college so I want to get as many in as I can. All the phone calls after football games and text messages before the games were so meaningful to me. I hope that over these 18 years of my life that I have made you proud. I know I'm not the brightest, most athletic or best all around but I have tried my best to make you proud and represent you with integrity and honor. You have taught me many things in life both on and off the field. You taught me how to be a man of respect. You taught me how to treat women the right way. All of my moral values come from you. You taught me how to always play fast and physical. You have contributed to my burning passion for sports. I will never forget the times when we would watch sports and talk about the Braves. You have raised me the right way, you have never forced or pressured me to do things I'm not comfortable with. It's hard to believe that all these moments have led to this. But I wouldn't do it any other way or with a better father. I will love you forever Dad. With much love from your son. Love Jack Burke."

This next letter was written to me in 1st quarter 2015 when I was attending a CRHP retreat at St Brigid in Johns Creek, GA. "Dad, When I heard you attending this retreat I was extremely happy and proud of you. Over the years you have consistently become stronger and stronger in your faith. You have been a great role model for me in this way. I strive to be strong in my faith like you. I have read a number of articles that talk about college students losing their faith or straying away from their core values. Because of you, I have continued to practice Catholicism at a university, surrounded by others, who question my beliefs. I have resisted temptations by relying on my core values that you taught me as a young man. In Deuteronomy 6:6-9 it says, "These commandments that I give you today are to be upon your hearts. Impress them on your children. Talk about them when you sit at home and when you walk along the road, when you lie down and when you get up. Tie them as symbols on your hands and bind them on your foreheads. Write them on your doorframes of your houses and on your gates." You have instilled the Lord's words and commandments into Allie and I. In times of trouble, I can turn to my faith and you as a father for guidance and help. I am truly grateful for that, and I am excited to continue growing my faith with you.

You have mentioned about mistakes in the past, but everyone including myself has made mistakes. The great thing about mistakes is that we made mistakes in the PAST. The past can no longer be changed so we are able to learn from them and move on. 1 John 1:9 says "If we confess our sins, he is faithful and just and will forgive us our sins and purify us from all unrighteousness". The Lord is so forgiving! Mistakes are in the past and the future is bright because of the Lord. Trust in him, and the plan he has made for you.

Dad you have been a huge supporter in my life in everything. Whether it be faith, grades, football, girls or whatever, you have always been there. I'll never forget the game against Western Carolina as I was being carted off. I was terrified, numb and scared. I was immobilized on the stretcher not able to look at anyone or sit up. It was completely silent and then I heard you say "everything is going to be alright Jack." It may have seemed so small in the moment but it resonated with me and I'll never forget it. You provided me with strength, at that very moment. I hope I can provide you with strength as we continue our journey through. You are a great father and man. Thank you for all you have done, your current support and the future support I know you will give. I would like to leave you with the quote I wrote on my wrist during the Samford games. Joshua 1:9 says "Be strong and courageous. Do not be terrified, do not be discouraged, for the Lord your God will be with you wherever you go." I love you Dad. Jack.

Chapter 7
Rediscovery

I used to go to 7:30 a.m. mass every Sunday at Saint Brigid Catholic Church in Johns Creek, Georgia. When Jack was in college, we went to the church together whenever he visited me over the weekend. At his mom's house, he would call me up and say,

"Dad, I'm coming home this weekend. Can I meet you at 7:30 a.m. mass? And afterward, we can get breakfast."

It made me very happy.

When I was at Georgia Regional Hospital in the fall of 2017, I fell asleep watching TV in the common area while sitting in a chair. As a result, I pinched a nerve and couldn't use my left hand for three months. It was paralyzed.

It took me a whole weekend, but I successfully filled out the Social Security disability application right-handed. I am left-handed for writing and eating and playing sports right-handed; I'm ambidextrous. And after three months, I gained full use of my left hand and wrist again. Initially, I thought I had a stroke.

I received one-year probation for the original misdemeanor charge of trespassing and terroristic threats against my neighbor in Forsyth County. In addition, I paid $47 per month for a year that ended in November of 2020 for the felony assaulting charge in Forsyth County jail; I received five-year probation for a first-time offender, and that probation was terminated in November 2020 after two years and two months.

When I was unemployed, I would go to Dr. Munjal, and he would give me $1,200 worth of Geodon samples because I didn't have insurance, and before, it went to generic.

So a month's supply of my medicine was $400.

Another thing I was able to accomplish while on my medicine and after getting my guardianship and conservatorships terminated was fixing my mailing address. I called Social Security and had then changed my address to my current address in Alpharetta at the Extended Stay America hotel because all my communication with Social Security was sent to my sister Betsy. I also contacted Fidelity (they manage my Pfizer pension).

I had previously tried to contact them to find out if they had offered me a lump sum money amount, and they would not speak to me because my sister had guardianship and conservatorships over me. I couldn't believe it, and I even asked my sister if she knew anything about that, but she never responded. I even sent her an email in February 2022:

Dear Betsy,

I hope all is well and you find a job soon. Life presents challenges, but I hope you got the rosary and gift card I sent you for Christmas. I'm shocked you never sent me an acknowledgment text. Let me say again I appreciate you packing up my clothes and furniture, buying me clothes while I was in the hospital, and also for visiting me in jail and at the Georgia Regional Hospital.

Mom told me yesterday that Dr. Browning told you I wasn't a nice person while I was at Georgia Regional Hospital. I yelled at Dr. Browning when I was first admitted. I was psychotic and angry after spending a year in jail and being mistreated by the guards. I didn't trust Dr. Browning and thought he was part of a conspiracy to mistreat me.

I couldn't understand why Dr. Browning was always so mean to me even as I got better and I spent much longer time in Georgia Regional Hospital unnecessarily. When I first arrived there, I truly enjoyed it when you visited, but that all changed when I hired Tom Ford.

Then after I got out of the hospital, you were so hard to communicate with. You wouldn't give me all my money, and you never offered me to stay with you when I needed it. So I went to New York with Tommy because I had no money, no credit, and nowhere to stay.

When I asked for my money to buy a car, you waited over a month before you sent me any, and then you restricted how much you would send.

I didn't get the remaining balance of my money until two years later, when I moved back to Georgia. Even though I asked for it multiple times to pay off my debts and hire an attorney to get my guardianship and conservatorship terminated.

While I was in jail, you recommended that Michael get guardianship and conservatorship from me. You rejected the thought of paying my mortgage, which was only $1,060 per month after Sam contacted you with the mortgage company info, and she has told me you weren't interested. The enormous amount of money you spent on attorneys to get guardianship and conservatorship from me could have easily been spent getting my mortgage current with plenty to spare.

To this day, you still don't respond to my texts and rarely did when you controlled my rights. You didn't even have the decency to show up in court when I had my rights restore hearing. But thanks for at least sending an attractive attorney, which ultimately I had to pay $4K for. She was nice to me.

While in jail, I never would have needed to hire Daisy Weeks to defend me when you took me to court to get guardianship and conservatorship from me, which cost me over $9.6K. You even said on the stand nasty and awful things about me, and I even had to endure Allie and Cheryl doing the same thing while I was psychotic, observing all of it, but I remember. Do you have any idea how that made me feel?

Also Tommy said he offered to go to my house and live there and pay my mortgage while I was in jail, but you rejected that.

Do you even remember when I went to your apartment in New York and rescued you from Mike, your abusive and druggy boyfriend? I gave you a place to stay for a few days at my home in New Jersey while you found a new place to stay. Even though you weren't really invited, I even welcomed you and Mike to my home in Chicago during Jack's Christening. I was trying to keep Cheryl happy.

Since coming back to Atlanta, I've been to therapists, and more than once told me I should be mad at you.

I don't hate you, Michael, Allie, or Cheryl. I've forgiven all of it, and I am ready to get reconnected. I'm still in pain from everything, but I know God will guide me and protect me.

Love always,

Unfortunately, she never got back.

Pfizer bought out Warner Wellcome, with whom I worked for eleven years. So that is why they hold my pension. It is a blessing, though; I'll be able to count on that money in retirement. So now I can freely call Pfizer, and they have advised me on how to proceed.

From February 1, 2023, I will be making approximately $900 a month in my pension.

In my mental health journey, I am a huge advocate for mental health hospitals and medicine. After everything I've gone through, all the heartache and loss that I have experienced, I truly believe in the value and help mental health hospitals offer. Through this book and my experience, I hope that people will learn more and empathize while also educating the criminal justice system about handling and treating prisoners with mental health problems more fairly and quickly. There is no way that I should have been allowed to stay in jail for one full year without receiving any medicine or any medical treatment whatsoever.

I would like to thank attorney David Rogers, the public defender handling my Johns Creek misdemeanor. He was very sympathetic to people with mental illness, as his brother has one. I received one-year probation but never had to report or pay any fees. My Forsyth County misdemeanor charges were $47 per month, and I had to report monthly by mail remotely for one year. That probation ended in November 2019.

I would like to thank my psychiatrist, Dr. Arun Munjal, originally from India. He is a real nice man and a great doctor. I've been seeing him since 2002, bimonthly for years. I should never have decided to go off my medicine in January 2015. Dr. Munjal told me not to, but I didn't listen to him.

I was convinced that my medicine was causing weight gain, high triglycerides, and high blood pressure. I used to see him when I was unemployed, and he only charged me minimal fees and also gave me samples.

While I didn't have insurance, I even tried to get medical coverage once when I was unemployed and had the money to buy insurance, but I got denied because of a pre-existing condition.

I don't know if that says we have a health care problem in this country, but the bottom line is we do, and we live where people can't be treated for mental health easily and quickly when they are incarcerated or get in trouble with the law or even lose a job.

On Christmas Eve in 2014, my sister Betsy planned to come over to the house to spend Christmas Eve and Christmas together. She was going to spend the night. I was always grateful to have family close by because I always got lonely during Christmas. I would see my children and celebrate Christmas, but it was always before or after the actual holiday.

My sister Betsy is single, and I was single, and it was great having her company. I felt very confident back then because I made $98,000 a year working in business development with SAP, and I started exercising at the gym on the treadmill and doing some weight work.

Betsy ended up coming over to the house four hours late. When she arrived, she was very rushed, and I confronted her about why she was so late. She got angry and very defensive, and soon enough, we got into an argument. She got angry and then threw her purse at me. Finally, she lit up, stormed out of the house, and went home. I felt awful about it and wanted to do something to make it up to her.

Every Christmas, I used to fill stockings for my children, Allie and Jack, and Betsy on the mantle in the family room. So what I did on Christmas Day, the next day, I drove down to her condo in midtown Atlanta and delivered the stocking contents at her concierge desk. I asked the receptionist to give her a note.

I was hoping that was a gesture to let her know how sorry I was for the argument. I was on my medicine then. When I went to see Dr. Munjal and told him about the episode with my sister, he recommended that he increase the dose of my medicine. However, I disagreed with him.

The following is everything I accomplished since moving back to the Georgia and Alpharetta area in May 2020. First, I successfully asked my sister Betsy to send me the remaining balance from my lump-sum payment from Social Security disability.

I used that money to pay off the remaining debt I had incurred while incarcerated at Forsyth County jail and Georgia Regional Hospital. The next thing I had to focus on was getting my guardianship and conservatorships terminated.

I had hired Mandy Moyer from Georgia probate lawyers in December of 2019. She agreed to represent me and initially petitioned the court on my behalf. But unfortunately she had to stop representing me because my sister's lawyer objected to her representation since she used to work for the judge in a probate court in Forsyth County.

Mandy told me she could fight it, but it would just cost me more money in attorney's fees in court time. I initially paid her $3,250, and she ended up returning a portion of that money.

So then, after moving back to Georgia, I started the process of finding a doctor to evaluate me and fill out an affidavit telling the court that I no longer needed a guardian or conservator. I had the most challenging time finding a doctor.

I called one doctor in Alpharetta, and she recommended that I contact the doctor that took my insurance, and she said I needed to have a complete psychological evaluation. So finally, I got a doctor in Dacula, GA, about forty-five minutes away. She agreed to do a psychological assessment for me.

Shirley Boone Sanford is a psychologist. I did the four-and-a-half-hour evaluation at the end of July of 2020. And the reports were completed and given to me on September 9, 2020. According to Georgia law, I needed two doctors to vouch for me and fill out an affidavit telling the court I no longer needed a guardian or conservator.

The following person to contact was my longtime psychiatrist, Dr. Arun Munjal. Even after all those years of seeing Dr. Arun and being stable on the medicine again after going off it in 2015, I have taken my medicine every day since September of 2017.

While being at Georgia Regional Hospital, I had been on the medication for nearly four years, so there were no symptoms of psychosis and no paranoid behavior, and it was like I never had the illness. So the medicine works that well.

Dr. Munjal wanted to see the evaluation done by Shirley Boone Sanford before he agreed to fill out the affidavit on my behalf. When I first saw him, I approached him about it, and he said he wanted to wait six months before he filled out the affidavit. So it wasn't until November 20, 2020 that he could successfully fill out the testimony on my behalf and get it notarized.

He even told me how hard it was to find a notary to get it notarized, and I had to pay him an extra $150, but he had to pay the bank notary that he used, all because of the pandemic. So I then submitted Dr. Munjal's and Shirley Boone Sanford's affidavit to the court and petitioned the court to terminate my guardianship and conservatorships.

When I submitted the paperwork, I think I made an error, and the probate court judge at that time rejected my petition. He cited the reason was the petition was submitted incorrectly. When I went back to the court, I talked to the clerk, and the judge said they would still use both Dr. Munjal and Shirley Boone Sanford's affidavits, and all I needed was to find one more doctor and resubmit the petition. So I was now back to looking for a doctor to vouch for me one more time.

I knew I could also use a therapist, and I thought to use Constance, the therapist that I saw in 2014 and 2015. She saw me while I was on the medicine and while I was off the medication while employed at SAP. She was kind and agreed to work on my behalf.

The court asked me to submit the doctor's name to them, and they would send the final evaluation form and paperwork directly to her and give her instructions on how to fill out the affidavit and return it to the court. I had one appointment with Constance and submitted her name to the court. After that, Constance wanted to see me for a few appointments before she filled out the paperwork, which was entirely appropriate and understandable.

However, the court rejected Constance Cromartie as a valid therapist because she is only a licensed professional counselor. According to Georgia law, I could use any medical doctor, including a licensed clinical social worker, but not a licensed professional counselor. So I then was back to square one. Thankfully I asked Constance if she knew of any licensed clinical social worker who could help me.

She recommended Stephanie Robbins, close by in Alpharetta, a licensed clinical social worker. I called Stephanie, and she agreed to help me and see me, but she said she needed six appointments at $150 per appointment. Neither Constance nor Stephanie took my insurance. These were all out-of-pocket costs to me.

Stephanie completed her affidavit and submitted it to the court on January 15, 2021. Surprisingly at the same time, the existing probate court judge in Forsyth County unexpectedly retired due to sexual harassment allegations against him. The new Forsyth County probate court judge assigned was Daisy Weeks.

Daisy Weeks was the attorney public defender who initially represented me in the guardianship and conservatorship case. She even told me that usually, she only works on criminal matters, but she agreed to represent me. Also she did tell me that she didn't have a lot of experience in probate work.

Since Daisy Weeks was my initial attorney in the guardianship and conservatorship case, and now she is the new probate court judge, she excused herself from the case. The case was sent over to Forsyth County Superior Court Judge Bagley. He is the same judge who handled my felony charges. I successfully petitioned the court to terminate my felony probation in November of 2020 with the help of attorney Joseph Stauffer.

Forsyth County Superior Court Judge Bagley immediately reviewed my petition and decided that I needed legal representation for the final hearing, and he directed Mandy Moyer back to represent me now that he was the judge. Mandy was so kind to represent me. The final hearing was set, all the affidavits were already complete.

All Mandy had to do was show up to court and represent me. She did the legal work and successfully asked Stephanie Robbins to appear to court as a witness on my behalf, and I'm very thankful to Stephanie for doing so.

SCHIZOPHRENIA

In March of 2021, after a hearing in front of Forsyth County superior Judge Jeffrey Bagley, my guardianship and conservatorships were terminated.

All of my rights as a person and a citizen were restored. I was so happy; I had no idea how hard it was to do anything in your life financially or personally when someone else has guardianship and conservatorships over you. Very similar to Britney Spears's situation. Social Security wouldn't talk to me, and the person who manages my fidelity investments for my Pfizer pension wouldn't speak to me. My sister Betsy didn't talk to me either.

I couldn't vote in the 2020 presidential election. I researched it, and according to GA law, you cannot vote if someone has guardianship and conservatorship over you. My very attractive sister's female attorney, who attended the final hearing, did not dispute my petition to get the guardianship and conservatorships terminated. Betsy never showed up to the hearing, and I never communicated with her whatsoever.

At that time, my sister's attorney told me she was petitioning the court to have her attorney's fees paid for by me. At the time, I told her I disagreed with that because my sister wasn't disputing my petition. Betsy didn't need to have an attorney, to begin with. She already had my guardianship conservatorships.

Betsy's attorney's fees were $3,452.45.

Thankfully while at my final hearing for my guardianship and conservatorships termination petition, Judge Bagley told me later on that my sister's attorney brought up the interpleader case from my remaining house auction equity in his court as well. So I was able to get the case number.

And she told me that the remaining balance was over $102,000.00.

I initially thought Mandy Moyer would represent me in filing a petition to the Forsyth County Superior Court on my behalf in the interpleader case to get my remaining house money. However, after six weeks had passed, I contacted Mandy Moyer, and she informed me that she was not going to represent me in the interpleader case, and at that time, I decided I was going to do it on my own.

I even contacted Joseph Stauffer, the great attorney who represented me in the felony charge and then got my felony probation terminated, but he wasn't interested in this case. So what I decided to do was to go to the Superior Court clerk at Forsyth County with the case number in hand and ask her how I could file for a petition for a hearing to get in front of Judge Bagley.

She walked me through step by step early morning in the clerk's office, at the public computers, as I filled out the petition. It was easier than I thought. They had an area right there in front of the clerk's office with computers where you could fill out the petition electronically. It's amazing what you can accomplish if you overcome your fears of getting started and just going out and doing it.

I finally was able to get in front of Judge Bagley again to get the final task I needed to take care of after my whole ordeal and get the remaining house money from my house auction. My house was auctioned off because it didn't pay my mortgage for over a year while in jail in 2016 and 2017. The auction took place in June of 2017.

My sister got guardianship and conservatorship over me in July of 2017. The house was auctioned off for $267K, and my mortgage was $154K. At the time of the auction, most of the houses in my neighborhood were selling for $325K. So I showed up in court in front of Judge Bagley and the person representing the mortgage provider, who's from ALAW. He was a nice man.

There was approximately $102,000 remaining of house equity after the auction. The interpleader case was put before the court because many people asked to get part of that house equity money. Credit card companies, homeowners association, the state of Georgia tax Internal Revenue Service, probate court from Forsyth County, and the attorneys representing my sister.

At that hearing, Judge Bagley agreed for all the funds to be transferred to superior court Forsyth County and he released ALAW from all further responsibilities. He awarded ALAW about $1,800 in attorney's fees from the balance.

At that time, I asked Judge Bagley how I could retrieve the remaining amount of money distributed to me, and he said that I would have to file another motion with the court. As I was leaving the courthouse, I talked to the attorney from ALAW. He recommended that I not fight the decision to have my sister's attorneys paid and the money going to probate court Forsyth County.

He advised me to contact both of those attorneys representing them and file a joint motion in front of Judge Bagley. He said that would be the quickest way to get the remaining funds distributed to me. Needless to say, that was one great piece of advice.

I contacted the attorney for Forsyth County, Karen Pachuta of Jarrard Davis LLP, and the attorney representing bowling rice, my sister's attorney, Sam Bagwell. I told them that I was not going to contest their requesting funds from my house equity and that if we could file a joint motion, it would be the quickest way for them to get paid and for me to get paid.

They both agreed, and after a few phone calls, Karen Pachuta decided to file the joint motion, but we had to wait for Judge Bagley to review their individual petitions first before we filed the joint motion.

Without any new court appearances and with the collective action and the judge's order being pre-drafted and by Karen Pachuta, all Judge Bagley had to do was agree to it. The chief judge of the Superior Court of Forsyth County, George Jeffrey Bagley, signed the joint motion and order on August 4th, 2021. I picked up a check for $89,624.88 from Forsyth County on August 11, 2021.

My ordeal was finally over.

I now could focus.

I'm finishing my book and telling my story.

It took me many years to realize that I'm flawed and a sinner, and I need to work every day to be the best man that I can be to myself and others and ask for God's help. But I know deep down that I'm a good person and was a good dad to my children.

Chapter 8
SCHIZOPHRENIA—A WAY FORWARD

Throughout my time when I was off the medicine, as a full-blown paranoid psychotic, I had grievances and complaints about everyone and everything. I thought everyone was out to get me, but it wasn't true. I brought my own adversity upon myself due to my mental illness.

I know I was wrong to get off the medicine in the first place, and that not listening to anyone was also a horrible idea. I was feeling so good physically, of the medicine, while my mind was manic and acutely aware of everything, albeit mostly psychotic thoughts.

I didn't want to be considered mentally ill. In fact, for the most part, I deluded myself into thinking that I was fine and that all the people around me were wrong.

I only wish I knew and did better at that time. It was only when I started losing the support of people that I loved the most and saw my life crumbling, right in front of my eyes, that I could see past my misguided belief and that everything wasn't alright. I realized I needed help.

My life after the diagnosis of schizophrenia and before was entirely different. I changed and nurtured a lot during the process. My struggles defined me and sculpted me into the man I am today.

It ultimately brought me closer to God.

I have been an active advocate of therapies and medications for people with mental illness and their taboos. Mental illness is nothing but a chemical imbalance in the brain.

SCHIZOPHRENIA

I want to let each and every one reading this book, anyone suffering, know that there is always hope. Hold on to that hope and never give up. You are worth it, this is your life, and you deserve to enjoy it just like every other person does. Reach out to someone you trust or love. It can be anybody, your friends or family. If not, go to a therapist.

I would not have been the same person I am today without the assistance of Dr. Arun Munjal. I will always be grateful to him for his services and kindness. The role he played in my life was that of a guardian.

Schizophrenia is a deadly mental disorder that needs to be tended to immediately. It is characterized by displaying various symptoms such as delusions, hallucinations, disruptive speech, behavior, and impaired cognitive ability. And because there is no probable cure to it, it is best to get treated as early as possible to improve the chances of managing it.[1]

The treatment also depends on the symptoms and the intensity of the disorder. You might need to stay on medication for a long time, possibly even for life. There are various therapies people can opt for, just as individual psychotherapy, CBT (cognitive behavior therapy), and CET (cognitive enhancement therapy).[2]

Medications are always the last priority, but the psychiatrist might prescribe one or more based on your condition. From experience, I can assure you that having those medicines can save your life. Non-pharmacological treatments such as therapies should be used in addition to medications and not as a replacement.

The goal in treating schizophrenia is included targeting symptoms, preventing relapse, and augmenting the adaptive functioning so that the person can be introduced back as stable to the world. Even though the person might be on medications, the disruptive behavior may linger, so it is essential to carry on the non-pharmacological treatments.

---

[1] https://www.ncbi.nlm.nih.gov/pmc/articles/PMC4159061/
[2] https://www.webmd.com/schizophrenia/schizophrenia-therapy

Not only do these therapies ensure the stability of the mind and body, but they also fill in the gaps in pharmacological treatments. In addition, they look after the patient and make sure they adhere to the medications.[3] Patients who discontinue their medications are at a very high risk of relapse, leading to rehabilitation. Therefore, it is important to create general awareness and keep the patients informed about the intensity of their disorder.

Among the various therapies, maintenance treatment is essential to help prevent relapse. In addition to focusing on the patient, treatment programs also encourage family support and care, so there is a lower chance of relapse.

The symptoms of schizoaffective disorder, the form of schizophrenia I suffered from, vary from person to person. I suffered from paranoia and delusions. I had episodes of mania and mood swings.[4] Even though nobody forced me into getting treatment, I hated the thought of going to a psychiatrist. But in reality, it is the best thing to ever happen to me.

Now, for most of my life, I'm happy. I make $30.1K annually on Social Security disability. I currently live in a studio apartment. I have paid off all my debts. I have a 2016 SUV with 29,800 miles that is paid for and a pension that will start in February 2023 after I turn sixty-two. I will make an extra $900 a month with my pension from Pfizer, and I have $70K saved.

I want to find an affordable townhouse in the upcoming years, and I'll be working on that until I reach my goal. I walk five miles two to three days a week, weather permitting, and I'm averaging fourteen-minute miles at a time. I am also doing pushups and dumbbell workouts multiple times a week, averaging six sets of fifty pushups in an hour, hoping and trying my best to cut down my weight.

I haven't been this strong since I was married. I am six feet tall and currently weigh 225 lb.; managing my overeating has always been a problem. I was 200 lb. in April 2021. When I left prison and

---

[3] https://www.ncbi.nlm.nih.gov/pmc/articles/PMC4159061/
[4] https://www.mayoclinic.org/diseases-conditions/schizoaffective-disorder/symptoms-causes/syc-20354504

went to Georgia Regional Hospital, I was 158 lb. I lost 61 lb. after one year in jail. At Georgia Regional Hospital, after getting back on mental health medicine, I gained 47 lb. back and weighed 205 lb. at discharge after one year in September 2018.

Going to the sacrament of confession is like therapy with God. That is the brilliance of the Catholic Church. I wish I had embraced that sacrament more when I was married.

The Catholic Church teaches forgiveness. Therefore, by writing this book, I hope to earn forgiveness from my ex-wife, Cheryl, and be friends with her again. Also, I want to re-establish the relationship I had with my kids and earn their love, respect, and forgiveness. I hope that I can be a part of their lives once again.

In summary, one of the reasons I felt comfortable hanging out with women escorts, women at massage parlors, and women at strip clubs was because I was craving female companionship. They were so friendly and welcoming to me. They didn't judge me for having a mental illness.

Of course, the interactions were transactional in nature, but when I talked to them, they actually listened to me and were very accommodating. They were willing to explore what I felt as I sought affection and intimacy. I just felt loved.

I would like to find that kind of affection now, with a woman for a relationship. I didn't feel like I was doing anything wrong. I didn't judge, and neither did they. I know it's probably not the right behavior, but that is how I felt about it at the time. The reality is, I'm just a very lonely man and crave female affection and love. I function much better when there is a woman in my life. I've always been that way.

It took me many years to realize that I'm flawed and a sinner. I need to work every day to be the best man that I can be for myself and others and constantly ask for God's help. I know deep down that I'm a good person, and I was a good, and loving father to my children.

I started writing this book based on a recommendation by Dr. Munjal and my former therapist, Constance Cromartie. They both encouraged me to write a book about schizophrenia in an attempt to help educate people so more people can understand the illness.

It is my hope that after this book is published and more people read it, mentally ill patients and prisoners are dealt with care, concern, and patience by law enforcement authorities. I hope some changes can be made to laws in Georgia that help the incarcerated get mental health assistance more rapidly when they go through any legal process.

From my earliest days in high school, all I ever wanted in life was to be a loving husband and a good, caring father. The good Lord gave that to me once, and then the damned schizophrenia took it away.

Perhaps that was what God had planned for me. He wants me to thrive and learn from what life offers. I curiously await what he has planned for me presently and also for my future. But I know, for now, my pain has softened and I hope for the best.

Please, Lord, guide me!

I would like to share a prayer I recently learned while attending a wonderfully powerful silent retreat at Ignatius House, a Jesuit retreat center. It is St. Ignatius Loyola spiritual exercise #234.

Take, Lord, and receive all my liberty, my memory, my understanding, and my will—all I have and possess. You, Lord, have given all that to me. I now give it back to you, O Lord. All of it is yours. Dispose of it according to your will. Give me love of yourself along with your grace, for that is enough for me.

Chapter 9
LESSONS LEARNED

Some of the things that I have learned since being back on my medicines and being stable is that I am a person who constantly needs validation in every aspect of my life. I need to know whether I am doing the right thing or not. I believe I always performed very well personally and professionally when I had a woman in my life towards whom I could focus my efforts. I crave intimacy and love from a woman, to put it right.

When I was married to Cheryl and was in love with her, all I wanted was for her to be happy, and I did everything to make her happy. I wanted to earn money so we could have a better life for ourselves and our wonderful children. When I met Cheryl in college, I was a beer-drinking frat boy, and I met her at the very end of my junior year.

I communicated with her all summer via letters that I mailed to her, and when I came back to campus after the break, I couldn't wait to resume seeing her and get a relationship with her.

We dated for a few weeks, but then she told me she wanted to break up and gave another guy a shot, someone she got to know over the summer. I thought she was a great girl, very beautiful, and I also thought she was too good for me. She was smart, and during that short dating duration, I stayed out of trouble. I wasn't drinking as much with my buddies and focused on hanging out with her. When she asked me to break up, I was hurt to the core.

But then, there was a two-way dance with my fraternity and her sorority. We hung out and drank, and we ended up dancing together.

And I ended up passionately kissing her on the dance floor. She then told me she wasn't seeing that guy anymore.

I was happy to resume our relationship. A lot of my friends and frat buddies couldn't believe we were dating. It was because I was nice to her after we broke up, I never talked bad about her, and I was always friendly to her because that is how I thought I would win her back.

She told me she was so happy that I was so nice to her even though we had broken up and that was one of the main reasons why she wanted to date me again.

Long story short, we dated my entire senior year. To give some context of how important she was to me, I had taken up eighteen credit hours during the fall of my senior year, which is one more class over the normal course load. In the spring, in order to graduate in April and not have to stay over and take a class during summer school.

I took twenty-one credit hours, i.e., seven courses, to graduate on time. I even had to get special approval from Dean Hoben of the University of Dayton Business School to take that many classes in one semester. And I passed all my courses. Between those two semesters, I scored a 3.0-grade point average in my senior year.

They made up for the terrible grades I got during my sophomore year when I was partying and hanging out with the wrong people. My two older brothers graduated in four years, and I was determined to as well. I wouldn't have been able to do it if it wasn't for Cheryl.

Even when I was married to Cheryl, I always wanted to make her happy. I gave her all of my salary and even the bonus money with which she paid all the bills. We made joint decisions on big purchases because she was always good with money, and I just wanted her to love me. It worked out pretty well.

My career was blossoming. I was getting promoted and transferred, and we were shifting from smaller houses to bigger homes, and then when we moved to Atlanta. I switched jobs to work for Coca-Cola. I thought we had made it. We had $1,000,000 in the bank. We had a beautiful home, two beautiful kids, a boy and a girl, and we were all very happy.

We both were making good money and after some time, she even started making more money than me. But I didn't care; I just wanted more of her time and intimacy.

Schizophrenia derailed all that, and you've read my story. Even after my divorce, I didn't start doing well until I started to date Sam exclusively. When I started to focus on seeing her more and pleasing her, my life came into focus. I was going to church. I was so excited to see Sam when we got together.

I fell in love with her. She was good for me in my professional life as well. I stopped going to strip clubs. I wasn't going to massage parlors. My business career blossomed when I got the job with SAP.

The lesson I've learned with schizophrenia is that you need to work out and exercise a lot. On the medicine, you tend to gain weight. And I've always had a problem with overeating. When I'm active, walking, doing pushups, I feel good about myself physically.

In the past, I mistreated my body for overeating and smoking since my divorce. Now, I have to stay focused and treat myself better. The lesson I've learned is that I have to stay with this medicine for the rest of my life.

I'm a happier person. It makes me a better candidate to be a future husband. I've always focused my life on pleasing others—the woman in my life, my children, customers at work, and colleagues and managers at work. I hope I can reunite with my children one day, and I'm so grateful that I still have my spiritual life at St. Brigid Catholic Church. It is amazing after all the things that happened to me, my church St. Brigid and the pastor, Fr. Neil Herlihy, welcomed me back with open arms, despite one of the parishioners from whom I was trying to rent a furnished apartment, and he was afraid to rent to me when he found out I had schizophrenia.

It just shows how some of the stigma having a mental illness puts on you in today's society. The illness has severed my relationship with my sister Betsy, my children, and my ex-wife, Cheryl.

One day, Sam and I met as I was walking; it was just out of the blue, and she was driving by and saw me. It was as if God brought her back into my life. She told me I look really good and asked for a hug and said, "We had a lot of fun together." That made me feel loved and appreciated. I still have lingering feelings for her, but she is married now, and I wish her the best and only want her to be happy in her life.

I'm grateful for the time we spent together and how she helped me focus on my life and get the job with SAP. Unfortunately, it didn't work out with Sameitria, but there are always future women that I hope the good Lord will bring into my life.

Well, I've learned since I moved back to Georgia from New York, and I am constantly trying to improve myself and deal with setbacks. If I handle my binge eating and continue with my exercising, I'll get the body I'm looking for, and I'll be more healthy.

I have set a goal for myself to be one hundred and eighty pounds. Everything will fall into place if I get there, and I'll be attractive enough to find a wife. And I will once again have a woman in my life to focus on to motivate me to be the best man that I can possibly be.

It has been a long road back, but through the grace of God as of June 9, 2022, I moved into a one bed one bath 800 Sq ft apartment in Peachtree Corners, GA. With great sidewalks only one mile from the Town Center and the Forum, with outstanding entertainment and shopping, only fifteen minutes from my church, St. Brigid. Peace Be With You All!

About the Author

An all-people loving Catholic man who values kindness and the goodness of all God's people.

CPSIA information can be obtained
at www.ICGtesting.com
Printed in the USA
LVHW051519140623
749623LV00002B/369

9 781662 487187